Alex Mold · Peder Clark ·
Gareth Millward · Daisy Payling

Placing the Public in Public Health in Post-War Britain, 1948–2012

Alex Mold
Centre for History in Public Health
London School of Hygiene & Tropical Medicine
London, UK

Peder Clark
Centre for History in Public Health
London School of Hygiene & Tropical Medicine
London, UK

Gareth Millward
Department of History
University of Warwick
Coventry, UK

Daisy Payling
Department of History
University of Essex
Colchester, UK

https://doi.org/10.1007/978-3-030-18685-2

Acknowledgements

The research that forms the basis of this book was conducted as part of a Wellcome Trust Medical Humanities Investigator Award held by Dr. Alex Mold. The project, 'Placing the Public in Public Health: Public Health in Britain, 1948–2010', grant number WT 100586/Z/12/Z, was based in the Centre for History in Public Health at the London School of Hygiene and Tropical Medicine (LSHTM). The project was made up initially of four strands and each was the primary responsibility of one member of the team. The strands and staff were: the place of the public in health education and health promotion (Alex Mold); health surveys, public opinion and the public's health (Daisy Payling); chronic disease, with a focus on coronary heart disease (Peder Clark); and infectious disease, with a focus on vaccination (Gareth Millward). A fifth strand, on public health and emotion (Hannah Elizabeth), was later added to the project, but the research from this work came too late to feature in this book.

Like the project on which it is based, this book is very much a collaborative endeavour. Alex Mold took the lead in framing the book and the chapters, and the main body of the book was written together. The fact that this was a relatively smooth process is a testament to the team, but also to the support we received from a number of key individuals and institutions. Hannah Elizabeth has been this book's best 'critical friend', pushing us and our work in exciting new directions. Ingrid James has supported us in making this research happen and resolved innumerable practical problems with exemplary calm. Our other colleagues in the Centre for History in Public Health, especially Virginia Berridge, Martin Gorsky, Chris Sirrs, John Manton, Hayley Brown, Erica Nelson, Janet Weston, Sue Taylor, Mateusz Zatonski, Ros Stanwell Smith and Anne Hardy have been hugely helpful, providing advice and guidance throughout the duration of the project. We were also supported by our project advisory group, the members of which included Professor David Evans from the University of the West of England; Professor Sally Sheard from the University of Liverpool; the archives team at the LSHTM and Erin Lafferty, the School's Public Engagement Coordinator.

Away from the LSHTM, we are grateful to the audiences at the conferences and seminars where members of the team spoke about this research. There are too many to list in detail here, but special thanks to audiences at the Society for the Social History of Medicine conferences in Oxford, Kent and Liverpool; the European Association for the History of Medicine and Health conference at Lisbon and Bucharest; and the meetings of the NHS 'tribe' of Wellcome funded projects on similar topics at the universities of Warwick and Liverpool. These meetings were particularly helpful in enabling us to speak to researchers working on similar themes but in different places and contexts.

Archives and libraries remain essential to the work of the contemporary historian. We would like to thank the staff at the National Archives, the British Library, the Wellcome Library and Archives and the library and archives staff at the LSHTM.

We are grateful to the history publishing team at Palgrave, especially Molly Beck and also to Tom Crook who provided insightful comments on the manuscript.

All of us have been supported by family and friends during the research and writing of this book. There are simply too many people to name—but you know who you are!

Finally, we would like to thank the Wellcome Trust, not only for the grant that allowed this research to happen, but also for being a supportive funder throughout the research process.

Contents

CHAPTER 1

Introduction

Abstract The Introduction sets out the key questions to be explored, summarises the main arguments and describes the case-studies used to consider these issues in depth. What was the place of the public in public health in post-war Britain? How did this change over time, and why does this matter? We briefly describe how we go about answering such questions by introducing the reader to our case-study areas. These are: the changing nature of health education; the public health survey; the response to heart disease; and the development of vaccination policy and practice. We also set out what each chapter will cover and argue.

Keywords The public · Public health · Public health history

In July 2006, the Labour Prime Minister Tony Blair gave a speech on healthy living. He began by stating that 'Today I focus on what we call "public health" but which is really about "healthy living"'. Blair went on to set out the challenges to public health as he saw them. He asserted that 'Our public health problems are not, strictly speaking, public health questions at all. They are questions of individual lifestyle - obesity, smoking, alcohol abuse, diabetes, sexually transmitted disease'. Whose responsibility, Blair pondered, was it to deal with such problems? The answer, he argued, was that 'Government should play an active role in the way the enabling state

A. Mold et al., *Placing the Public in Public Health in Post-War Britain, 1948–2012*, Medicine and Biomedical Sciences in Modern History,
https://doi.org/10.1007/978-3-030-18685-2_1

should work: empowering people to choose responsibly'. Indeed, Blair went on, 'in many cases government is not the organisation to persuade us to change some of our most personal behaviour. So Government needs to work with others - with industry, with the media, with civil society to have an impact on persuading more people to make more healthy choices'. The public's health, the Prime Minister suggested, was the responsibility of individuals, the state, and private and voluntary organisations.

Blair's speech offers a particular vision of how public health problems and solutions were seen in Britain in the early twenty-first century. But the speech is also interesting because of how it uses history. Blair contrasted the public health problems of the contemporary period with those of the mid-nineteenth century. He suggested that the 'big state' was needed to deal with epidemic disease and poor living conditions. State action was still required to combat the public health problems of today, but, Blair argued, the purpose of the 'enabling state' was 'to empower the individual', in contrast, he argued, to 'command and control in the manner of 1945' (Blair 2006). Historical example was being used to justify an apparently new view of the relationship between the state and citizen, between the public and public health policy and practice. In this book, we explore the extent to which this shift took place, and the reasons for it. We contend that the place of the public in public health changed over time, but much depends on the meaning of 'the public' and of 'public health'. Neither of these entities were fixed categories, and as understandings of publics and their health shifted, so too did ideas about the rights and responsibilities of the state and its citizens.

The standard interpretation of this shift is the one exemplified by Blair's speech: during the second half of the twentieth century, as public health problems became linked to individual behaviour, greater emphasis was placed on personal efforts towards securing good health. Historian Dorothy Porter argued that 'By the end of the twentieth century states facing the inexorable rising costs of providing health services from increasingly aging and chronically sick populations transformed personal wellness into an individual contribution to the commonwealth' (Porter 2011, 2). State action was still needed, but the 'new public health' required a new kind of citizen: one that lived in a prudent and vigilant way to guarantee their good health (Petersen and Lupton 1996). For some, the notion of this 'entrepreneurial self' threatened the 'publicness' of public health by individualising and privatising risk (Petersen 1997).

While there is much to be said for this narrative as a way of characterising the broad changes around public health from the nineteenth century to the present, we want to complicate the story. By analysing the changing meanings of the public and of public health in post-war Britain, we suggest that while notions of 'the public' encountered individuating forces, such as the rise of identity politics and risk factor epidemiology, 'the public' as a collective continued to matter. For instance, we will show that although there were tensions between individual rights and collective responsibilities surrounding population and personal health, most of the people most of the time accepted an ongoing duty to safeguard their own health and that of others. 'Publicness' in a larger sense, as a set of values, collective spaces, services and actions, retained a sense of importance for both the state and the citizenry. Moreover, not all of the changes to understandings of the public and public health were imposed from above. We draw attention to some of the ways in which the public, or rather certain publics, had agency and were able to 'speak back' to public health policymakers and practitioners, although some had more agency than others.

Indeed, it is clear that there was not one 'public' but many 'publics', as well as various ways of seeing these.

In this book, we get to grip with the nature of some of these publics and the scenarios in which they were created. To do so, we draw on our historical research, which has examined the place of the public in public health in Britain from the establishment of the National Health Service in 1948 to the 'return' of public health services to local government in 2012. Through this work, we present a new perspective on the relationship between state and citizen in the post-war period. Based on the papers of key organisations, government records, published sources and oral history interviews, we explore the dynamics of public-public health interaction in four areas. We focus on the changing nature of health education; the public health survey; the response to heart disease; and the development of vaccination policy and practice. These examples were selected as they encompass the key technologies and techniques of public health practice and research, as well as some of the main challenges to population and individual health. Analysing the response to chronic conditions like coronary heart disease, and the ongoing efforts to deal with vaccine-preventable infections, allows us to see how changes in patterns of disease and its aetiology influenced the relationship between public health and the public. Looking at the methods by which public health policymakers, researchers and practitioners addressed the public, through the survey and in health education campaigns enables us to explore the ways in which public health authorities conceived of the public. We are also able to use these sources to think about how various publics used these media to 'speak back' to public health. This allows us to see the public not as an inert or passive object only to be acted upon, but as a dynamic entity in possession of its own agency.

1 Outline of the Book

The concepts of 'the public' and 'public health' have been subjected to a range of interpretations and definitions over time. In Chapter 2, we consider historical and theoretical approaches to both 'the public' and 'public health'. Neither concept has a fixed meaning, but by tracking some of the key formulations of each, we point to both change and continuity over time. Indeed, one of the constants is the fluidity of 'the public', which was never one thing, but many. Similarly, 'public health' encompasses a variety of projects, subjects and objects. We bring clarity to such a complex picture by sub-dividing 'the public' and 'public health' into categories. 'The public' can be seen firstly, as a collection of people; secondly, as a space for action; and finally, as a set of values. In a similar vein, 'public health' can be broken down into a set of different parts. We describe 'public health' as consisting of the challenges it faced or faces; the systems employed to deal with these; and finally, as a philosophy or outlook. To show how these worked in practice, and also to set our research in context, we also use Chapter 2 to present a brief overview of the changing nature of the relationship between the public and public health from the nineteenth century to the early twenty-first century.

The precise nature of the 'public' being imagined in post-war Britain is the topic of Chapter 3. In this chapter, we point to three ways in which public health policymakers and practitioners perceived the public. The public was sometimes seen as a collective, as a mass or the entire population. But this mass public was often broken up into groups, many of which aligned with well-established tropes, such as class, gender and ethnicity. Members of the public were also envisaged as individuals. Such neat categories were far from rigid and in this chapter we also point to instances when imaginings of the public overlapped or even conflicted with one another. For public health practitioners, the imagined public was never an entirely coherent entity.

In Chapter 4, we probe the nature of the public in more depth, specifically by turning things around and looking at how the public 'spoke back' to public health. We point to three modes of speaking back: resistance, complaint and reappropriation. Resistance could be 'active', like refusal to participate in a particular public health initiative, or 'passive', like being reluctant or hesitant to engage. Complaining about public health policies or practices, as with complaining within healthcare in general, was rare, but complaints offer a valuable insight into the concerns of the public. Indeed, some members of the public were able to go a step further, and reappropriate or re-ascribe meaning to particular public health messages. All of this indicates that the public was not a passive actor within public health in the post-war period.

The extent to which notions of 'the public' and 'public health' changed over time are alluded to throughout the book, but in Chapter 5 we interrogate this issue in more detail. Here we return to the question posed by Tony Blair in his speech in 2006: what was the role of the public in safeguarding its own health, and what was that of the state or other actors? We point to ways in which 'the public' was challenged by 'private' interests and factors as well as how it was reinforced. The linking of many chronic conditions to individual behaviour undoubtedly had an impact on the operation of public health as a practice, as a set of services, and as a philosophy. Individuals and their conduct were always important, but now they mattered more than ever. This undermined some elements of what had been 'public' about public health in the past, but, we argue, there was also a range of new ways in which 'publicness' was retained and even remade in the latter decades of the twentieth century. At the same time, there was also a plethora of other developments beyond the public/private dichotomy that nonetheless had an impact upon notions of the public and its health.

The changing relationship between public health and the public offers important insights into the nature of publics, public health and publicness in post-war Britain. In Chapter 6, we reflect on changes and continuities in the place of the public, the nature of public health and the relationship between these. We relate these developments to understandings of citizenship. In this way, we contend, the specific case study of the place of the public within public health has much to teach us not only about publics, their health and the people and systems that are supposed to safeguard this, but also about the interaction between state and citizen.

Bibliography

Blair, Tony. 2006. 'Speech on Healthy Living.' 26 July. http://webarchive.nationalarchives.gov.uk/+/http:/www.number10.gov.uk/Page9921.

Petersen, Alan. 1997. 'Risk, Governance and the New Public Health.' In *Foucault, Health and Medicine*, edited by Alan Petersen and Bryan Turner, 189–206. London and New York: Routledge.

Petersen, Alan, and Deborah Lupton. 1996. *The New Public Health: Health and Self in the Age of Risk*. London: Sage.

Porter, Dorothy. 2011. *Health Citizenship: Essays in Social Medicine and Biomedical Politics*. Berkeley and Los Angeles, CA: University of California Press.

CHAPTER 2

The Public and Public Health

Abstract In this chapter, we explore conceptualisations of the public, of public health and the relationship between these. We suggest there are three key ways in which 'the public' is seen: as a collection of people; as a space for action; and as a set of values. Likewise, public health can be understood in terms of: the challenges it faced or faces; the systems employed to deal with these; and as a kind of philosophy or outlook. We also look at the changing nature of the relationship between the public and public health. We begin in the nineteenth century, move on to the early twentieth century, and map out the broad elements of the dynamic surrounding public health and the public after 1945.

Keywords The public · Public health · Public health history · Population · Citizenship · Public sphere

Who or what is the 'public' in 'public health'? How have these concepts changed over time, and what impact does this have on the relationship between the public and public health? In this chapter we set out to address these critical questions. We argue that the 'public' and 'public health' are not fixed or concrete entities: these are constructions that alter over time and place. The slipperiness of such concepts makes them hard to define, but by studying their malleability, important aspects of the nature of the

A. Mold et al., *Placing the Public in Public Health in Post-War Britain, 1948–2012*, Medicine and Biomedical Sciences in Modern History,
https://doi.org/10.1007/978-3-030-18685-2_2

social and political action that surrounds collective and individual health are revealed. For instance, it is often the case that there is not one 'public' but many 'publics'. A single, unitary public may have rhetorical value, but the practice of public health tends to encompass a range of publics. Likewise, although 'public health' in its literal sense as the 'health of the public' might appear to be a stable object, it is a moving target shaped by a range of forces, systems and ideas.

In this chapter, we seek to untangle some of these complexities through an exploration of theoretical and historical perspectives on the public, public health and the relationship between these. We begin by examining the concept of 'the public'. The public, like 'the nation' or 'the masses' is a construct, and there are, we suggest, three key ways in which 'the public' is seen. Firstly, as a collection of people; secondly, as a space for action; and finally, as a set of values. After exploring each of these in turn, we analyse the notion of 'public health'. Different definitions of public health will be examined, and by reflecting on how these have changed over time, we identify three core components. Public health can be seen in terms of: firstly, the challenges it faced or faces; secondly, the systems employed to deal with these; and finally, as a philosophy or outlook. In the final section of the chapter, we look at how the relationship between the public and public health in Britain has changed over time. We begin in the nineteenth century, move on to the early twentieth century, and map out some of the broad elements of the dynamic surrounding public health and the public in the post-Second World War era. Developments from the late 1940s onwards will be interrogated in more detail throughout the rest of the book, but it is important to both set the scene and think about how continuities and changes in publics and public health play out over the *longue durée*. This reiterates our argument that both the public and public health are multiple and ever-changing, but it also helps to point out when, where and why such changes may have occurred.

1 The Public

'The public', like other grand organising concepts such as 'the nation', or 'the masses', is imaginary. As the legal scholar John Coggon points out, the notion of 'the public' has much in common with Benedict Anderson's concept of imagined community. No member of the public can know all the other members of the public, but in their minds or those of others they are part of one community (Coggon 2011). Similarly, drawing on Raymond

Williams's analysis of the 'masses', the historian David Cantor notes that there was no such thing as 'the public', only ways of seeing it (Cantor 2002). What is meant by the 'public', according to social policy analysts Janet Newman and John Clarke, is often 'elusive' (Newman and Clarke 2009, 11). Some critics have even suggested that 'the public' is too ambiguous a term to be of use (Mathews 1984, 122). Yet, the concept is employed frequently, and in many contexts, so it clearly has value. Analysing the ways in which the concept of 'the public' is mobilised helps provide useful insight into its meanings. As Coggon and Newman and Clarke indicate, 'the public' exists simultaneously as an object and as a descriptive, normative category. We can see how this works in practice by considering the ways in which 'the public' operates within definitions of public health. Marcel Verweij and Angus Dawson identify two 'senses' of the public within public health. The first relates to the state of the health of the public, the population or the collective. The second revolves around a set of interventions aiming to protect the health of the public. The public is thus a thing to be targeted and a process of collective action (Verweij and Dawson 2007). This is useful but leaves out a sense of the values attached to the concept of 'the public'. As Newman and Clarke argue, part of what makes the public is a set of legal and democratic values that mark out a domain distinct from private interests (Newman and Clarke 2009, 4).

From these different descriptions of 'the public' we derive three sets of meanings of the public that deserve further analysis. Firstly, the public as the people, citizens and/or the population; secondly, the public as a space for action, intervention and service provision; and finally, as a set of collective values, often, but not always, opposed to private interests. These groups of meanings reflect the different senses of the public discussed in the literature but also take us beyond it, towards thinking about how 'the public' is deployed in specific contexts and how this changes over time.

1.1 Public = Population, Citizens

'The public' is often seen as synonymous with the 'population' or the 'citizens' of a place. Populations and citizens are not the same entity, but they are related concepts as they both refer to the public as a noun. The notion of the 'population' is particularly relevant here, as it is bound up with the history and practice of public health. The collection and collation of statistics about life and death that began in Britain as early as the seventeenth century was crucial to the development of knowledge about the public and its health (Porter 1999, 5, 49–52). The Annual Reports of the Registrars-General running from 1839 to 1973, and today's equivalent Office for National Statistics publications, were an essential resource for headline data on mortality, and, by extension, endemic and newly emergent diseases. These ways of viewing the public, based on assumptions of distribution of data and probability, are essential to both public health's epistemological roots and its scientific credibility.

Yet, the population was more than a statistical product. As Tom Crook and Glen O'Hara point out, the generation of numbers about the public enabled them to be imagined in new ways (Crook and O'Hara 2011). The social epidemiologist Nancy Krieger argues that in addition to the common understanding of population as a statistical entity defined by innate attributes, populations are also dynamic, defined by relationships among their members and with other populations (Krieger 2012). Like 'the public', 'population' is relational (Cantor 2002). This can be seen when the uses to which this concept is put are examined in more detail. For followers of Foucault, population was a product of bio-political power: coming to know the population was essential to governing it (Foucault 2007). What the sociologist David Armstrong termed 'surveillance medicine' brought everyone—sick and well—into the purview of public health authorities (Armstrong 1995). The generation of data about the population and its health was essential to its improvement, but also to the expansion and development of public health as a practice and a philosophy. Attempts to improve population health and develop the systems to do so were a crucial part of the formation of the modern state (Szreter 2003; Porter 1999; Crook 2016; Hamlin 2010).

Population, however, was not the only way in which states envisaged the people in relation to health or other spheres. Notions of citizenship were fundamental to states and their government from Ancient Greece onwards (Heater 2004, 2006). Yet, the concept of what it meant to be a citizen changed considerably over time, especially surrounding the rights and responsibilities of states and citizens. As Dorothy Porter notes, public health in the nineteenth century was concerned with protecting citizens from epidemic diseases (Porter 1999, 63–96, 111–46). By the early twentieth century, ideas about social citizenship came to the fore. These emphasised the provision of public services, like healthcare, as part of the social contract between state and citizen (Marshall 1992). The post-war establishment of the welfare state in Britain, and particularly the NHS, is often seen as the apogee of social citizenship. For Porter, this was dictated by a social, rather than economic logic, one that justified intervention from the state to achieve national efficiency and improved public health. Closely related to the concept of social medicine, social citizenship emphasised a medicine of society for society (Porter 2011, 113–24). Social citizenship, according to Harry Oosterhuis and Frank Huisman, meant that healthcare was a right not a favour (Oosterhuis and Huisman 2014).

From the 1970s onwards, however, social citizenship and the entitlements it encompassed came under threat. The rising costs of healthcare, coupled with the growth of neoliberalism, and the apparent increase in incidences of lifestyle-related disease, provoked a new formulation of health citizenship. What Oosterhuis and Huisman term 'neo-republican citizenship' emphasised civic responsibilities and obligations in relation to health. They argue that neoliberal ideas about the value of market models of healthcare provision and the importance of individual choice and autonomy combined with a 'new public health' that placed the responsibility for managing public health risks squarely on the citizen rather than society (Oosterhuis and Huisman 2014). Yet, as Porter remarks, there was still a role for the state in the provision of healthcare and intervening in the social and political environment to allow citizens to achieve better health (Porter 2011, 113–24). We examine the changing nature of health citizenship in greater detail throughout the book, but it is worth noting that whatever notion of citizenship held sway, this was not all-encompassing. As Matthew Grant comments in his survey of formulations of citizenship in post-war Britain, certain groups of individuals were often excluded from the notion of British citizenship and, at the same time, citizens themselves could engage with ideas of citizenship to make it their own (Grant 2016). When viewed as either populations or citizens, the public was not merely a passive actor.

1.2 Public = Space for Action

The capacity for the public to act compels us to think about the spaces in which it acts, or is acted upon, and what these actions involve. 'The public' can be regarded not just as an object, but also as a space for action. One of the principle ways of viewing this surrounds the notion of the public sphere. The chief architect of this concept is the German theorist Jurgen Habermas. Beginning in the late seventeenth century, Habermas charts the development of new forms of bourgeois sociability related to the rise of capitalism (Habermas 1989). In places such as coffee houses and salons, and through other mechanisms like the popular press, a separate space distinct from the state and the private realm began to emerge (Calhoun 1992; Sturdy 2002). This space, which Habermas characterised as the 'public sphere', allowed individuals to debate collectively issues of wider significance. Yet, almost as soon as it began to emerge, the public sphere came under threat. As the public enlarged beyond the bourgeoisie, particularly through the extension of the franchise to the working classes, and capital and economic power became concentrated in the hands of the wealthy, the public sphere became riven by competing interests. The state had to intervene to mediate such conflicts, resulting in the public sphere and the state becoming ever more interlinked. The distinction between state and society, and between the public sphere and the private sphere, broke down. As a result, instead of being concerned with rational debate, the public sphere became the site of negotiation between interest groups. Once the bourgeois public became a mass public, participation in the public sphere was reduced to a plebiscite with the power to direct state action and limited to simple voter approval or disapproval.

Developing Habermas's theory, Craig Calhoun contends that the enfranchisement of the working classes in the nineteenth century and women in the early twentieth century, followed by the rise of identity politics in the latter half of the twentieth century, fractured the unified public sphere, leading to the creation of multiple or overlapping public spheres (Calhoun 1992). The notion of a single public no longer held weight, according to Nancy Fraser, as even subordinated groups were able to come together to form 'subaltern counter publics' (Fraser 1990). The literary scholar Michael Warner contends that there was nothing 'subaltern' about some of these counter publics: they set themselves up in direct opposition to 'the public' and offered alternative ways of thinking about the nature of public life (Warner 2002a, b). Once again, the literature suggests that not only are there multiple publics but that these exist in relation to one another and sometimes in opposition to dominant formulations of 'the public'.

Habermas's theory of the public sphere, influential though it is, is not the only way of thinking about how the public is enacted. The other key space for action surrounds what is done for, or in the name of, the public. This encompasses many areas, but the most relevant here is the provision of public services. As Newman and Clarke note, public services are 'both constituted by, and constitutive of, notions of publicness' (Newman and Clarke 2009, 4). Public services help shape publics (and vice-versa) in multiple ways. For instance, public service bodies act as channels for public culture. In their study of the BBC in Britain during the 1980s, Patricia Holland, Hugh Chignell and Sherryl Wilson explore the nature of public service broadcasting and how it dealt with the public (Holland 2013). They suggest that during this period, notions of public service shifted away from a paternalistic understanding of the public as clients and towards a more libertarian view of the public as consumers. Underpinning this was a change in the ideals attached to publicness. The public then, is not just about actors and action, it is also about values.

1.3 Public = Values

The values ascribed to publicness are often described in relation to what the public is not. The most common juxtaposition is public versus private. A set of binaries revolve around different conceptions of public and private. Public is often taken to mean collective, whereas private refers to the individual. Or it can be a set of spaces: private relates to the home, public to the spaces outside it. Within public health practice, there have long been tensions over the distinction between the public and the private realms. In the nineteenth century, the development of legislation around sanitation and the cleansing of environments encroached upon private spaces as well as public ones (Daunton 1990). Other kinds of public health initiatives, such as vaccination, were seen by some to impinge upon the private body of the individual and their right to determine what happened to it (Durbach 2005). A further reconceptualisation of the boundary between private and public was implicated in the rise of lifestyle-related disease, as what might previously have been thought of as private matters, like drinking and smoking, came to be seen as public health dangers.

In the context of healthcare and other welfare services, 'private' can also mean market-orientated or for profit, while 'public' describes state-funded or supplied forms of healthcare. Values are often attached to these binaries. For some, public services, like the NHS, are an inherent good which needs defending against the incursion of private interests (Pollock 2005). Others argue that public service providers may not always act in the best interests of individuals and that private, market-orientated modes of working would be more efficient and effective (Le Grand 2003, 2007). In this book, we do not attempt to arbitrate between such opposing views, rather we point out where these tensions exist and explain how they came into being.

One long-running trend associated with the values connected to publicness is a fear that the public is in decline. The American sociologist Richard

Sennett outlined 'the fall of public man' from 'his' [sic] height in the eighteenth century to a 'state of decay' by the time of writing in the mid-1970s. For Sennett, it was the bleeding together of private and public realms, especially around feelings and sentiments that were previously confined to the private sphere, that brought about decline (Sennett 1977). Approaching this from a rather different perspective, Nikolas Rose argues for the role of psychology and other 'psy' disciplines in creating private selves, but for Rose there are other influences too, such as biomedicine and biotechnology which help 'make up' (borrowing from Ian Hacking) 'biological citizens' (Rose 1999, 2006, 2010; Hacking 2006). For other commentators, the growing importance being ascribed to individuals was the flip-side of the demise of collective ways of thinking about people and their interests. David Marquand outlines what he sees as the 'hollowing out' of the public domain in Britain since the 1970s. Marquand contends that the cultural revolution of the late 1960s and 1970s helped to break down distinctions between the public and the private as the personal became political. At the same time, economic crisis opened the door to neoliberal attacks on collective welfare systems. The deregulation and privatisation of public services that took place from the 1980s onwards, Marquand asserts, 'narrowed the public domain and blurred the distinction between it and the market domain' (Marquand 2004, 2).

Despite such elegies for the public, the extent to which the public can be said to have declined depends on the values which are ascribed to it. As Newman and Clarke point out, there are all sorts of ways in which 'publicness' is retained and even remade within contemporary public services (Newman and Clarke 2009). Efforts to increase public participation in public services, for instance, have proliferated in recent decades (Stewart 2016; Hogg 2009; Baggott et al. 2005). 'The public' is still a concept that does work, even if the nature of this work may have changed over time. This can be seen when we broaden the discussion away from 'the public' and think about 'public health'.

2 Public Health

Describing the nature of 'public health' is just as problematic as outlining that of 'the public'. Historian Christopher Hamlin points out that 'The great debate in the history of public health is what public health is and what it should be' (Hamlin 2011, 411). The very process of defining public health is a normative exercise, and one which has changed over time.

Nonetheless, in their survey of a series of definitions of public health from the 1920s onwards, Verweij and Dawson identify two common elements. Firstly, public health is about the state of the health of the public, that is the population, the whole or the collective. Secondly, public health encompasses interventions or practices that are aimed at protecting the health of the public. These interventions are not primarily those of an individual, but involve some form of collective action (Verweij and Dawson 2007). A much-used definition of public health is that put forward by the American bacteriologist CEA Winslow in 1920. He stated that public health is:

> the science and the art of preventing disease, prolonging life, and promoting physical health and efficiency through organized community efforts for the sanitation of the environment, the control of community infections, the education of the individual in principles of personal hygiene, the organization of medical and nursing service for the early diagnosis and preventive treatment of disease, and the development of the social machinery which will ensure to every individual in the community a standard of living adequate for the maintenance of health. (Winslow 1920)

Many contemporary definitions of public health draw on Winslow's, but the elements that get removed and added are often telling. The historian Virginia Berridge cites two definitions of public health in UK government reports, one from 1988 and one from 2004. Both reports use the formulation of public health as the 'science and art of preventing disease, prolonging life and promoting health through the organised efforts of society', but the 2004 definition adds 'and informed choices of society, organisations, public and private, communities and individuals'. Berridge ascribes the difference in definitions to the widening range of actors involved in ensuring that population health be improved and the changing politics of what 'public health' is thought to encompass (Berridge 2016, 3–4).

The politics of defining public health is also explored by Coggon. He identifies 'seven faces of public health'. First, he suggests, public health is a political tool. Public health is used as a compelling reason for formulating a policy. Second, public health is a business of government. Public health is a government function, whether that relates to specific agencies or governmental powers that affect health. Third, public health operates as a social infrastructure; it can be used to describe a society's organisation with respect to health issues. Fourth, public health is a professional enterprise. Fifth, public health can be used as a qualifier to represent probable benefits or harms within a population. Sixth, public health is a moral enterprise: any member of the public may do harm or benefit to the others through their actions. Finally, public health is the population's health; it is the health of the population either in aggregate or by distribution (Coggon 2011). These seven faces are useful, but for our purposes a little unwieldy. Instead, we group ways of defining 'public health' around three core sets of meanings. Firstly, public health has often been understood in relation to the challenges that face population health. Secondly, public health can be described as a set of systems. Finally, public health can be thought of as a philosophy or outlook.

2.1 Challenges

Public health is often shaped by the issues it contends with. Just as the issues have changed over time, so too has the meaning of public health. As Porter remarks, for many, the history of public health 'conjures up an image of investigating toilets, drains and political statutes through the ages' (Porter 1999, 1). Although public health in the sense of what Porter calls 'collective action in relation to the health of populations' has existed for centuries, a particular type of 'public health' that developed during the nineteenth century, and was connected to sanitation and the state, tends to dominate conceptions of 'public health' in the past (Porter 1999, 4). Such conceptions can pose problems when thinking about more recent formulations of public health. Jane Lewis asserts that 'While the focus of nineteenth-century public health seems clear, writers have found it hard to describe the content of public health in the twentieth century' (Lewis 1986, 5). Lewis suggests that after the Second World War public health 'allowed itself to be defined by the activities is undertook. The idea of public health thus remained indistinct' (Lewis 1986, 3). We get to grips with this argument in more detail later in the book, but for now it is worth surveying briefly the different types of challenges that were defined as public health problems, and how these shaped conceptions of 'public health' at various times.

The nineteenth century was a period when concerns about the impact of sanitation and the environment on health dominated. This was the case in Britain, Europe and North America (Baldwin 2005; Nathanson 2007; Hamlin 2010; Rosen 1993). Endemic and epidemic infectious diseases such as cholera, typhoid, typhus and smallpox were the leading causes of morbidity and mortality. Political, social and economic pressures to combat these diseases resulted in the development of bureaucratic systems and technological fixes to fight infection. The building of sewers, the development of refuse collection, the provision of clean water, sanitary inspection, the introduction of vaccination, and so on, were all measures designed to protect and improve population health. By the early twentieth century, many infectious diseases appeared to have been conquered, as morbidity and mortality from these conditions decreased. The exact role played by public health initiatives in this is disputed (improvements in nutrition and the quality of housing were also important) but it is the case that by the early 1900s public health authorities began to shift their attention to other issues (McKeown 1979; Szreter 2002). Infant mortality and child health, tuberculosis and personal and social hygiene became key concerns (Welshman 2001; Niemi 2016).

As the incidence of infectious disease continued to decline throughout the twentieth century, the nature of what was meant by 'public health' also shifted. The diseases people suffered, and therefore the activities necessary to improve population health, changed. By the post-Second World War period, it appeared that an 'epidemiologic transition' had taken place (Omran 2005; Weisz and Olszynko-Gryn 2010; Armstrong 2014). Chronic conditions, such as heart disease and cancer, had overtaken infectious disease as the leading cause of death (Weisz 2014). From the mid-1950s, epidemiological studies began to demonstrate a link between individual behaviour and certain chronic conditions. The most famous of these concerned smoking and lung cancer, but other work also found connections between coronary heart disease and diet as well as levels of exercise (Doll and Hill 1950; Morris 1957). Such conditions and their aetiology seemed to pose a new type of challenge to the public's health and those that sought to safeguard it. Improving public health now involved persuading individuals to change their behaviour and thus decrease their chances of developing a chronic disease. What became known as 'lifestyle public health' focused on identifying and reducing 'risk factors' for chronic disease through health education and other preventive measures such as screening (Rothstein 2003; Oppenheimer 2006). By the end of the twenty-first century, the challenges facing public health were vastly different from those of 200 years prior, and so 'public health' as an enterprise was also altered.

2.2 *Systems*

To address collective health problems, a range of different systems were created at different times. Tom Crook, in his book on late nineteenth- and early twentieth-century public health describes public health 'systems' as: 'a shifting assemblage of interacting parts and practices, people and things' (Crook 2016, 3). These systems were complex and dynamic, and not necessarily 'systematic' in the sense of being methodical, but nonetheless their architects hoped that they would be. Within this broad definition of a public health system, Crook identifies a wide range of actors and authorities. These include central and local government and their agents, as well as other entities such as private companies and civil society. Although Crook is describing a period over 100 years ago, many of the same key actors can be identified throughout the recent history of public health systems. That is not to say that public health systems stay the same. Indeed, the nature of public health systems, and especially the location of public health services, altered over time. A key area of both continuity and change surrounds the relative role of central versus local government.

Since the introduction of key pieces of legislation such as the Public Health Act in 1848, the national government may have directed developments, but it was often local government that had to take action. The establishment of local Boards of Health, and the creation of the role of the Medical Officer of Health (MOH), put the onus on local government to develop public health services and systems. The duties of the MOH changed over time in line with the challenges facing population health. In the late nineteenth and early twentieth centuries these included sanitary inspection, vaccination, the collection of statistics on death and disease and directing improvements to housing. By the early twentieth century, according to Martin Gorsky, the MOH had reached the height of his (MOH were almost all men in this period) powers (Gorsky 2007). MOH had responsibility for (among other things) state welfare programmes to improve the health of children and mothers, school medical services, screening and, after 1929, the former Poor Law workhouses which operated as chronic disease hospitals. Some historians have suggested that during the inter- and post-war years MOH were ineffective and failed to adapt to the changing nature of public health problems (Webster 1988; Lewis 1986, 1991). Others have argued against this, pointing to individual MOH who were willing and able to deal with new and ongoing public health problems such as malnutrition (Gorsky 2008; Welshman 1997b).

Regardless of the effectiveness or otherwise of MOH, a key moment in the development of public health systems in Britain occurred at the time of the creation of the NHS in 1948. Some of the duties and responsibilities of MOH and local government, including the chronic disease hospitals, were transferred to the new health service. MOH had fewer services to administer, but they still had a role to play in areas such as disease prevention and health education (Diack and Smith 2002; Welshman 1997b; Mold 2018). Yet, some of these responsibilities were also shared with other agencies, including central bodies like the Ministry of Health and the Central Council for Health Education, and other local actors such as General Practitioners (Blythe 1987). Further change came after the NHS reorganisation in 1973–1974. Responsibility for public health was removed from local government and brought within the NHS. The post of the MOH was scrapped and replaced with that of the community physician. Integrating 'public health' services and functions within the NHS was supposed to make them more effective, but there were difficulties. The community physician worked within the local NHS structures to coordinate preventive services. Many community physicians struggled with their new role, attempting to balance health service management with planning and specialist preventive duties. It was also unclear what 'community medicine' meant, and what this empowered the community physician to do (Lewis 1986).

More recently, the location of public health services and functions in England (the situation is different in each of the devolved nations) changed again. Public health once more became the responsibility of local government following the Health and Social Care Act, 2012. Commissioning for public health services was moved out of the NHS and devolved to local government. Directors of Public Health were relocated to local authorities, where they oversee health protection and improvement in their area, as well as the provision of public health services such as smoking cessation, sexual health and drug and alcohol treatment (Gorsky et al. 2014). At the same time, central government and the NHS also retain some responsibility for public health, as well as a whole host of other agencies and actors. Clearly there is not one 'public health system': it is diffused and located in various places, and has been for decades. Yet it can be helpful to think about the myriad ways in which systems shape ideas about public health, and how ideas about public health shape systems.

2.3 Outlook

What distinguishes a 'public health system' from any other health system? In part, this can be attributed to the philosophy or outlook of the system and the people running it. Commentators often talk about a 'public health approach' to an issue, or the need to find a 'public health solution'. This can be seen, for instance, in relation to illegal drug use. In 2016, two leading public health agencies called on the UK government to reorientate drug policy towards improving and protecting public health rather than focusing on criminal justice (Royal Society of Public Health and Faculty of Public Health 2016). The emphasis on health protection and health improvement was no coincidence, as these are two of the three core functions of public health outlined by one of the report's authors, the Faculty of Public Health. Yet, as Berridge notes, the 'core functions' of public health are also influenced by the location of public health services (Berridge 2016, 6). Moreover, the existence of the Faculty of Public Health, as the standard setting body for public health practitioners, complete with qualifications, exams and membership, points towards the development of a public health 'profession'. The Faculty was established in 1972 following a recommendation from the Todd Commission on medical education. Yet the nascent profession was far from united. Lewis highlights considerable tensions between community physicians and academics, such as Jerry Morris, who wanted to ground public health practice more firmly in epidemiology (Lewis 1986, 102). This casts doubt on the idea that there was or ever could be a single 'public health view' of any given issue. Yet, certain elements have, over time, been associated repeatedly with a public health outlook or approach.

A key feature of a public health view is the emphasis on tracking and surveying health and illness at a population level. One of the roles of MOH and their successors was to gather and record statistics on the health of the people in their area. Epidemiology was central to the development of public health practice and public health research from the nineteenth century onwards. The nature of epidemiological theory changed over time, in line with patterns of disease and wider medical thought. There was, for instance, often tension between biological and social explanations of disease causation and its spread (Krieger 2014). However, one constant surrounds the need to explain the distribution of disease within the population. Obtaining the data to analyse the causation and spread of disease required an element of population surveillance. Some scholars, especially those influenced by Foucault, see this as one of the methods by which public health authorities exercise power over the population. Armstrong, for instance, argues that the development of surveillance medicine in the early twentieth century expanded public health's gaze to include the entire population, pathologising the normal as well as the abnormal. Alan Petersen and Deborah Lupton contend that this trend persisted with the development of the 'new public health' of the post-war era. They argue that 'Epidemiology is thus one of the central strategies in the new public health used to construct notions of "health" and, through this construction, to invoke and reproduce moral judgements about the worth of individuals and social groups' (Petersen and Lupton 1996, 60). Public health, they suggest, is not just a set of initiatives designed to improve population health, but also a moral enterprise.

Evidence for the ways in which public health practice and research is bound up with morality is certainly not difficult to find. There is a long tradition within public health of blaming the victim, of pathologising individuals (or groups of individuals) rather than focusing on the social conditions that give rise to incidences of disease. This can be seen in nineteenth-century attempts to blame epidemics of infectious disease on the poor; in early twentieth-century efforts to focus on bad motherhood as a cause for infant mortality; or in late twentieth-century health education campaigns which stigmatised the individual (Hamlin 2010; Apple 1995; Marks 1996; Lupton 2014). But, public health practice also has a counter-vailing tradition which emphasises social justice (Hamlin 2010). Again, this has been present since at least the nineteenth century, and although it was rarely dominant, the importance of social, economic and political structures in accounting for patterns of disease was not totally ignored. One element underpinning these conflicting views are contrasting notions of the place of the public in public health. How has the public been thought of within public health, and how has this changed over time?

3 The Changing Relationship Between Public Health and the Public

As we suggested in the Introduction, surprisingly little attention has been devoted to examining the nature of the relationship between the public and public health. Here we briefly survey the limited historical literature on this issue, focusing on three key periods: the nineteenth century; the early twentieth century; and the post-war period. Throughout these eras there was never a monolithic concept of either the public or public health, or a fixed relationship between them. 'The public' was construed in different ways and it interacted with a 'public health' that was constantly changing. Nonetheless, certain continuities can be detected. There has long been a role for the public within public health, even if the nature of this public, and its ability to affect change, was often constrained.

3.1 The Nineteenth Century

Ideas about the place of the public in public health in nineteenth-century Britain were strongly influenced by broader conceptions of the individual and their rights and responsibilities. Anne Hardy observes that the freedom of the individual was always more important within the British liberal tradition than in other countries such as Germany, something which can be seen in the 1848 Public Health Act. The provisions contained within this key piece of legislation were voluntary, not compulsory. State regulation relating to the individual body was even more contentious, as in the case of the vaccination laws: compulsory vaccination failed partly due to public opposition. Hardy remarks that 'In terms of public health, the case of vaccination demonstrates that there was not one public but many, even before the concept of "public health" had been formulated' (Hardy 2013, 93). The multifarious nature of the public was also reinforced by the extent to which it was interwoven with the state. James Hanley examined petitions to Parliament in the period 1847–1848 for evidence of public reaction to the development of public health legislation. He found that the petitions garnered a large number of signatories. Most of these were male and middle-class, although Hanley suggests that there was some support from working-class organisations too. This led him to conclude that the public was overwhelmingly in favour of sanitarianism as encapsulated within the 1848 Public Health Act (Hanley 2002).

Deborah Brunton investigated public reaction to public health legislation at the local level. Focusing on Scottish cities, Brunton points out that sanitary reform represented a significant intervention into the lives of private citizens. The agencies of local government grew, she suggests, as a response to this. In this way, local government was part of the public sphere, not distinct from it. Brunton argues that private, public and government interests overlapped to the extent that 'the private world of the citizen and the public realm of governance flowed into one another' (Brunton 2002, 172). Crook offers a different perspective on the relationship between the public, the private realm and the state within nineteenth-century public health. Drawing on Foucauldian notions of surveillance, Crook examines the role of the public health inspector and suggests that everyone (the public, local government and the state) was involved in inspecting everyone else, all in the name of the public. He argues that 'Inspectors inspected the public and its representatives; in turn, the public and its representatives inspected inspectors and the administrative field of public health' (Crook 2007, 381). Crook suggests that not all inspectors were resented as unwelcome agents of red tape; some had the respect of their communities. Inspectors also investigated public complaints, which could be quite numerous (Crook 2016, 142).

The ability to complain, though limited, did offer the public some scope to 'speak back' to public health. More active opposition to public health measures, however, was rare. One of the few initiatives that did provoke resistance was vaccination. Nadja Durbach found that anti-vaccination movements included participation from the more 'respectable' working classes as well as middle-class reformers (Durbach 2000). There were also numerous disputes between local and national authorities, and between public health officials and councillors and rate-payers over specific public health initiatives, such as sewerage and water supply systems (Crook 2016). 'The public' did have agency, but the public being conceived of here was almost exclusively white, male and middle-class.

3.2 1900–1945

The changing nature of population health, and especially the impact of the epidemiological transition from infectious to chronic disease, helped to alter the way that public health authorities viewed the public. Armstrong suggests that instead of being concerned about the relationship between the public and the environment, public health was now interested in the relationships between people (Armstrong 1983). Diseases such as TB and VD were seen as being socially infectious: passed on by contact between individuals. As Porter points out, the development of social medicine meant that there was also interest in the impact of social structure on health and a desire to focus on the 'whole person' rather than just the 'sick man' (Porter 2011, 104–24). Both these trends meant that public health policy authorities began to recognise that improvements in health would not be achieved through technological fixes or enhanced service provision alone, but also through the actions of the public itself. As a result, in the early twentieth century, and especially in the inter-war period, public health practitioners increased their efforts to educate the public in practices intended to improve their health. This can be seen in the establishment of the Central Council Health Education (CCHE) in 1927, and the efforts of MOH at the local level to educate the public in matters such as personal hygiene and good motherhood (Blythe 1987; Gorsky 2007; Welshman 1997b). These efforts, according to Welshman, were also aimed at promoting a certain standard of morality and designed to enhance citizenship, as well as health (Welshman 1997a).

Although the public was deemed educable in some matters relating to health, there were other circumstances where public health practitioners thought the public could not, or should not, be reached. Elizabeth Toon notes that most of the British medical community in the inter-war period were opposed to cancer education. They believed that the public was so afraid of cancer that it made people irrational. Education was deemed counter-productive, as it would only foster 'cancerphobia' (Toon 2007). The emotional nature of the public was thought to be damaging in other areas too. Cantor, in his study of the Empire Rheumatism Council, found that the medical men that made up the organisation during the 1930s saw members of the public as emotional, ignorant and unable to manage their own urges. It was only by monitoring and directing the emotional currents within the public that the public could be motivated to act in its own best interest. Cantor argues that up until the Second World War, the public was seen as an undifferentiated mass, but after this period the public began to fragment. He contends that the establishment of the NHS, the development of consumerism, and the application of epidemiological categories and scientific techniques began to break up the 'general public' into different groups (Cantor 2002). The extent to which this represented a true fragmentation of ideas about 'the public' is questionable, but this was a time when the public came to matter to public health in new ways.

3.3 Post 1945

Public health did not exist in a vacuum. Broad social, political, and economic change had an impact on public health practice and how it regarded the public. Over the course of the second half of the twentieth century, new ways of thinking about groups and individuals came to the fore. Social and political action surrounding gender, ethnicity, and sexuality gave rise to the creation of new identities. These new categories existed alongside and interacted with both each other and older notions of social class (Rosen

2003; Harris 2003). Indeed, class did not go away as a framing device or as an identity, although it did change as patterns of work, housing and family life also shifted (Savage 2008, 2015). For some critics, the growth of identity categories played a part in the demise of collective ways of seeing people (Marquand 2004). At the same time, the needs, wants and desires of individuals were increasingly prioritised by politicians. The General Election of 1979, and the establishment of the Conservative government under Margaret Thatcher, is often seen as a pivotal moment. The pursuit of a series of policies by Thatcher and her successors, from the right to buy council houses to the creation of an internal market within the NHS, emphasised the ability of individuals to improve their own circumstances. Shaped by neoliberal ideas of the primacy of the market, citizens were increasingly thought of as 'consumers' (Bevir and Trentmann 2007).

The history of consumerism encompasses both individual desires and collective needs (Hilton 2003). Indeed, it was initially hoped that consumerism could empower groups and individuals who had often been ignored. From the 1970s onwards, there were calls for greater public involvement in public services. Consumer bodies were set up within the nationalised industries, and national consumer groups, like the Consumer Council attempted to speak for consumers across the public and private sectors. In health, Community Health Councils (CHCs) were created in 1974 to be the 'voice of the consumer' within the NHS (Mold 2015; Hogg 2009). Although the record of organisations like the CHCs in affecting change was patchy, the citizen-consumer voice could not be ignored. CHCs were scrapped in 2003 and were replaced with an 'alphabet soup' of organisations with varying acronyms and short life spans (Mold 2015, 159–61). Nonetheless, the principle of public involvement within the NHS and other public services is now well-established, even if it is of questionable impact.

Alongside such wider shifts, changes in patterns of disease within the population also served to alter perceptions of the public. From the 1950s onwards, the linking of chronic conditions such as lung cancer to behaviours like smoking had a profound impact on the way in which public health authorities saw the public. A whole host of individual behaviours, including diet, exercise and alcohol consumption were shown to result in sickness and death. What Morris termed 'ways of living' shaped not only individual health and well-being, but health on a collective level too, as these were prevalent throughout the population (Morris 1957). To address these issues, public health authorities had to appeal to individuals. As Porter remarks, 'The key to the social management of chronic illnesses – such as lung cancer – was individual prevention raising health consciousness and promoting self-health care' (Porter 2011, 207). By the twenty-first century, she asserts, there is still some emphasis on the importance of social structure, social conditions and the environment on health, but health is now seen primarily as an individual responsibility (Porter 2011, 2002). This could, and indeed has, led some to argue that there is now no such thing as 'public' health, or at least that it no longer means what it did in relation to collective well-being (Le Fanu 1999; Fitzpatrick 2002). But, as this chapter has made clear, there have been and continue to be multiple ways of viewing the public and its health.

4 Conclusion

The multiplicity of 'the public' and 'public health' is one constant in a shifting story across time and place. By thinking about 'the public' as people, as a space for action, and as a set of values, we have shown that this dynamic concept can be put to a variety of uses. Additional complexities occur when we look at 'public health' and the elements that have defined it as more than just a description of death and disease at a population level. 'Public health' is shaped by the challenges it faced or faces, the systems employed to deal with these, and also a specific kind of outlook. Moreover, all these elements interact in different ways and at different times. There is no simple or single answer to the questions we posed at the outset of this chapter. Such complexity, should not, however, defy exploration or even explanation. Despite elegies for 'the public' and for 'public health' neither of these have gone away. Rather, they have been remade. In the rest of the book we explore how and why.

Bibliography

Apple, Rima D. 1995. 'Constructing Mothers: Scientific Motherhood in the Nineteenth and Twentieth Centuries.' *Social History of Medicine* 8 (2): 161–78.

Armstrong, David. 1983. *Political Anatomy of the Body: Medical Knowledge in Britain in the Twentieth Century*. Cambridge: Cambridge University Press.

———. 1995. 'The Rise of Surveillance Medicine.' *Sociology of Health & Illness* 17 (3): 393–404.

———. 2014. 'Chronic Illness: A Revisionist Account.' *Sociology of Health & Illness* 36 (1): 15–27.

Baggott, Rob, Judith Allsop, and Kathryn Jones. 2005. *Speaking for Patients and Carers: Health Consumer Groups and the Policy Process.* Basingstoke: Palgrave Macmillan.

Baldwin, Peter. 2005. *Contagion and the State in Europe, 1830–1930.* Cambridge: Cambridge University Press.

Berridge, Virginia. 2016. *Public Health: A Very Short Introduction.* Oxford: Oxford University Press.

Bevir, Mark, and Frank Trentmann. 2007. *Governance, Consumers and Citizens: Agency and Resistance in Contemporary Politics.* Basingstoke: Palgrave Macmillan.

Blythe, Max. 1987. *A History of the Central Council for Health Education, 1927–1968.* DPhil, University of Oxford, Green College.

Brunton, Deborah. 2002. 'Policy, Powers and Practice: The Public Response to Public Health in the Scottish City.' In *Medicine, Health and the Public Sphere in Britain: 1600–2000*, edited by Steve Sturdy, 171–88. London: Routledge.

Calhoun, Craig J. 1992. 'Introduction: Habermas and the Public Sphere.' In *Habermas and the Public Sphere*, 1–48. Cambridge, MA: MIT Press.

Cantor, David. 2002. 'Representing "the Public": Medicine, Charity and the Public Sphere in Twentieth Century Britain.' In *Medicine, Health and the Public Sphere in Britain: 1600–2000*, edited by Steve Sturdy, 145–68. London: Routledge.

Coggon, John. 2011. *What Makes Health Public? A Critical Evaluation of Moral, Legal and Political Claims in Public Health.* Cambridge: Cambridge University Press.

Crook, Tom. 2007. 'Sanitary Inspection and the Public Sphere in Late Victorian and Edwardian Britain: A Case Study in Liberal Governance.' *Social History* 32 (4): 369–93.

———. 2016. *Governing Systems: Modernity and the Making of Public Health in England, 1830–1910.* Oakland, CA: University of California Press.

Crook, Tom, and Glen O'Hara. 2011. 'The "Torrent of Numbers": Statistics and the Public Sphere in Britain, c. 1800–2000.' In *Statistics and the Public Sphere: Numbers and the People in Modern Britain*, 1–32. Abingdon, Oxon, and New York: Routledge.

Daunton, M. J. 1990. 'Housing.' In *The Cambridge Social History of Britain, 1750–1950*, edited by F. M. L. Thompson, 195–250. Cambridge: Cambridge University Press.

Diack, Lesley, and David F. Smith. 2002. 'Professional Strategies of Medical Officers of Health in the Post-war Period-1: "Innovative Traditionalism": The Case of Dr. Ian MacQueen, MOH for Aberdeen 1952–1974, a "Bull-Dog" with the "Hide of a Rhinoceros".' *Journal of Public Health Medicine* 24 (2): 123–29.

Doll, Richard, and A. Bradford Hill. 1950. 'Smoking and Carcinoma of the Lung.' *British Medical Journal* 2 (4682): 739–48.

Durbach, Nadja. 2000. '"They Might as Well Brand Us": Working-Class Resistance to Compulsory Vaccination in Victorian England.' *Social History of Medicine* 13 (1): 45–62.

———. 2005. *Bodily Matters: The Anti-vaccination Movement in England, 1853–1907*. Durham, NC: Duke University Press.

Fitzpatrick, Michael. 2002. *The Tyranny of Health: Doctors and the Regulation of Lifestyle*. London: Routledge.

Foucault, M. 2007. *Security, Territory, Population*. Edited by Arnold I. Davidson and Translated by Graham Burchell. 2009 ed. Basingstoke: Palgrave Macmillan.

Fraser, Nancy. 1990. 'Rethinking the Public Sphere: A Contribution to the Critique of Actually Existing Democracy.' *Social Text* (25/26): 56–80.

Gorsky, Martin. 2007. 'Local Leadership in Public Health: The Role of the Medical Officer of Health in Britain, 1872–1974.' *Journal of Epidemiology and Community Health* 61 (6): 468–72.

———. 2008. 'Public Health in Interwar England and Wales: Did It Fail?' *Dynamis (Granada, Spain)* 28: 175–98.

Gorsky, Martin, Karen Lock, and Sue Hogarth. 2014. 'Public Health and English Local Government: Historical Perspectives on the Impact of "Returning Home".' *Journal of Public Health* 36: 1–6.

Grant, Matthew. 2016. 'Historicizing Citizenship in Post-war Britain.' *The Historical Journal* 59 (4): 1187–1206.

Habermas, Jurgen. 1989. *The Structural Transformation of the Public Sphere: An Inquiry into a Category of Bourgeois Society*. Cambridge, MA: MIT Press.

Hacking, Ian. 2006. 'Making Up People.' *London Review of Books* 28: 23–26, 17 August.

Hamlin, Christopher. 2010. *Public Health and Social Justice in the Age of Chadwick: Britain, 1800–1854*. 1st Reissue ed. Cambridge: Cambridge University Press.

———. 2011. 'Public Health.' In *The Oxford Handbook of the History of Medicine*, edited by Mark Jackson, 411–28. Oxford: Oxford University Press.

Hanley, James G. 2002. 'The Public's Reaction to Public Health: Petitions Submitted to Parliament, 1847–1848.' *Social History of Medicine* 15 (3): 393–411.

Hardy, Anne. 2013. 'The Public in Public Health.' In *Beyond Habermas: Democracy, Knowledge and the Public Sphere*, edited by Christian J. Emden and David Midgley, 87–98. New York and Oxford: Berghahn Books.

Harris, Jose. 2003. 'Tradition and Transformation: Society and Civil Society in Britain, 1945–2001.' In *The British Isles Since 1945*, edited by Kathleen Burk, 91–125. Oxford: Oxford University Press.

Heater, Derek. 2004. *A Brief History of Citizenship*. New York: New York University Press.

———. 2006. *Citizenship in Britain: A History*. Edinburgh: Edinburgh University Press.

Hilton, Matthew. 2003. *Consumerism in 20th Century Britain*. Cambridge: Cambridge University Press.

Hogg, Christine. 2009. *Citizens, Consumers and the NHS: Capturing Voices*. Basingstoke: Palgrave Macmillan.

Holland, Patricia. 2013. *Broadcasting and the NHS in the Thatcherite 1980s: The Challenge to Public Service*. Basingstoke: Palgrave.

Krieger, Nancy. 2012. 'Who and What Is a "Population"? Historical Debates, Current Controversies, and Implications for Understanding "Population Health" and Rectifying Health Inequities.' *Milbank Quarterly* 90 (4): 634–81.

———. 2014. *Epidemiology and the People's Health: Theory and Context*. Oxford and New York: Oxford University Press.

Le Fanu, James. 1999. *The Rise and Fall of Modern Medicine*. London: Little, Brown.

Le Grand, Julian. 2003. *Motivation, Agency and Public Policy: Of Knights and Knaves, Pawns and Queens*. Oxford: Oxford University Press.

———. 2007. *The Other Invisible Hand: Delivering Public Services Through Choice and Competition*. Princeton, NJ: Princeton University Press.

Lewis, Jane. 1991. 'The Public's Health: Philosophy and Practice in Britain in the Twentieth Century.' In *A History of Education in Public Health: Health That Mocks the Doctors' Rules*, edited by Elizabeth Fee and R. M. Acheson, 195–229. Oxford and New York: Oxford University Press.

Lewis, Jane E. 1986. *What Price Community Medicine? The Philosophy, Practice and Politics of Public Health Since 1919*. Brighton: Wheatsheaf Books.

Lupton, Deborah. 2014. 'The Pedagogy of Disgust: The Ethical, Moral and Political Implications of Using Disgust in Public Health Campaigns.' *Critical Public Health* 25: 4–14.

Marks, Lara V. 1996. *Metropolitan Maternity: Maternal and Infant Welfare Services in Early Twentieth Century London*. Amsterdam and Atlanta: Brill and Rodopi.

Marquand, David. 2004. *Decline of the Public: The Hollowing Out of Citizenship*. Cambridge: Polity Press.

Marshall, T. H. 1992. 'Citizenship and Social Class.' In *Citizenship and Social Class*. London: Pluto Press.

Mathews, David. 1984. 'The Public in Practice and Theory.' *Public Administration Review* 44: 120–25.

McKeown, Thomas. 1979. *The Role of Medicine*. Oxford: Blackwell.

Mold, Alex. 2015. *Making the Patient-Consumer: Patient Organisations and Health Consumerism in Britain*. Manchester: Manchester University Press.

———. 2018. 'Exhibiting Good Health: Public Health Exhibitions in London, 1948–71.' *Medical History* 62 (1): 1–26.

Morris, J. N. 1957. *Uses of Epidemiology*. Edinburgh and London: E&S Livingstone.

Nathanson, Constance A. 2007. *Disease Prevention as Social Change: The State, Society, and Public Health in the United States, France, Great Britain, and Canada.* New York: Russell Sage Foundation.

Newman, Janet, and John Clarke. 2009. *Publics, Politics and Power: Remaking the Public in Public Services.* London: Sage.

Niemi, Marjaana. 2016. *Public Health and Municipal Policy Making: Britain and Sweden, 1900–1940.* Abingdon: Routledge.

Omran, Abdel R. 2005. 'The Epidemiologic Transition: A Theory of the Epidemiology of Population Change.' *The Milbank Quarterly* 83 (4): 731–57.

Oosterhuis, Harry, and Frank Huisman. 2014. 'The Politics of Health and Citizenship: Historical and Contemporary Perspectives.' In *Health and Citizenship: Political Cultures of Health in Modern Europe*, 1–44. London: Pickering and Chatto.

Oppenheimer, Gerald M. 2006. 'Profiling Risk: The Emergence of Coronary Heart Disease Epidemiology in the United States (1947–70).' *International Journal of Epidemiology* 35 (3): 720–30.

Petersen, Alan, and Deborah Lupton. 1996. *The New Public Health: Health and Self in the Age of Risk.* London: Sage.

Pollock, Allyson M. 2005. *NHS Plc: The Privatisation of Our Health Care.* New Updated ed. London: Verso Books.

Porter, Dorothy. 1999. *Health, Civilization and the State: A History of Public Health from Ancient to Modern Times.* London: Routledge.

———. 2002. 'From Social Structure to Social Behaviour in Britain After the Second World War.' *Contemporary British History* 16 (3): 58–80.

———. 2011. *Health Citizenship: Essays in Social Medicine and Biomedical Politics.* Berkeley and Los Angeles, CA: University of California Press.

Rose, Nikolas. 1999. *Governing the Soul: Shaping of the Private Self.* London: Free Association Books.

———. 2006. *The Politics of Life Itself: Biomedicine, Power, and Subjectivity in the Twenty-First Century.* Princeton: Princeton University Press.

———. 2010. *Inventing Our Selves: Psychology, Power, and Personhood.* Rev. ed. Cambridge: Cambridge University Press.

Rosen, Andrew. 2003. *The Transformation of British Life, 1950–2000: A Social History.* Manchester: Manchester University Press.

Rosen, George. 1993. *A History of Public Health.* Expanded ed. Baltimore: Johns Hopkins University Press.

Rothstein, William G. 2003. *Public Health and the Risk Factor: A History of an Uneven Medical Revolution.* Rochester, NY: University of Rochester Press.

Royal Society of Public Health and Faculty of Public Health. 2016. *Taking a New Line on Drugs.* London: Royal Society of Public Health.

Savage, Mike. 2008. 'Affluence and Social Change in the Making of Technocratic Middle-Class Identities: Britain, 1939–55.' *Contemporary British History* 22 (4): 457–76.

———. 2015. *Social Class in the 21st Century*. London: Penguin Random House.

Sennett, Richard. 1977. *The Fall of Public Man*. Cambridge: Cambridge University Press.

Stewart, Ellen. 2016. *Publics and Their Health Systems—Rethinking Participation*. Basingstoke: Palgrave Macmillan.

Sturdy, Steve. 2002. 'Introduction: Medicine, Health and the Public Sphere.' In *Medicine, Health and the Public Sphere in Britain: 1600–2000*, edited by Steve Sturdy, 1–24. London: Routledge.

Szreter, Simon. 2002. 'Rethinking McKeown: The Relationship Between Public Health and Social Change.' *American Journal of Public Health* 92 (5): 722–25.

———. 2003. 'The Population Health Approach in Historical Perspective.' *American Journal of Public Health* 93 (3): 421–31.

Toon, Elizabeth. 2007. '"Cancer as the General Population Knows It": Knowledge, Fear, and Lay Education in 1950s Britain.' *Bulletin of the History of Medicine* 81 (1): 116–38.

Verweij, M. F., and Angus Dawson. 2007. 'The Meaning of "Public" in "Public Health".' In *Ethics, Prevention, and Public Health*, edited by M. F. Verweij and Angus Dawson, 13–29. Oxford: Clarendon Press.

Warner, Michael. 2002a. 'Publics and Counterpublics.' *Public Culture* 14 (1): 49–90.

———. 2002b. *Publics and Counterpublics*. New York and Cambridge, MA: Zone Books and Distributed by MIT Press.

Webster, Charles. 1988. *The Health Services Since the War, Volume 1: Problems of Health Care, the National Health Service Before 1957*. London: HMSO.

Weisz, George. 2014. *Chronic Disease in the Twentieth Century: A History*. Baltimore: Johns Hopkins University Press.

Weisz, George, and Jesse Olszynko-Gryn. 2010. 'The Theory of Epidemiologic Transition: The Origins of a Citation Classic.' *Journal of the History of Medicine and Allied Sciences* 65 (3): 287–326.

Welshman, John. 1997a. '"Bringing Beauty and Brightness to the Back Streets": Health Education and Public Health in England and Wales, 1890–1940.' *Health Education Journal* 56 (2): 199–209.

———. 1997b. 'The Medical Officer of Health in England and Wales, 1900–1974: Watchdog or Lapdog?' *Journal of Public Health Medicine* 19 (4): 443–50.

———. 2001. *Municipal Medicine: Public Health in Twentieth-Century Britain*. 1st ed. Oxford and New York: Verlag Peter Lang.

Winslow, C.-E. A. 1920. 'The Untilled Fields of Public Health.' *Science* 51 (1306): 23–33.

CHAPTER 3

Imagining Publics

Abstract In this chapter, we examine how public health policymakers and practitioners imagined the public in post-war Britain. We focus on three ways of thinking about the public: as a whole or a mass; as groups; and as individuals. At the same time, these ways of imagining the public often overlapped and sometimes conflicted with one another. Moreover, public health practitioners' conceptions of the public interacted with pre-existing assumptions and values. This resulted in a fractured, but dynamic, sense of the public. Public health actors' conception of the public, we argue, was multifaceted, sometimes contradictory, and open to change over time. Part of what made public health 'public' was a continued interest in the collective as well as the individual or group.

Keywords Class · Gender · Ethnicity · Risk · Behaviour

In this chapter, we examine the various ways public health policymakers and practitioners imagined the public in post-war Britain. There were three key ways of thinking about the public. Firstly, the public could be seen as a whole, as a mass or as the entire population. Part of what made public health 'public' throughout this period was a continued interest in the collective as well as the individual or group. Secondly, the public could be broken up into distinct groups. Many of these fractured along familiar

A. Mold et al., *Placing the Public in Public Health in Post-War Britain, 1948–2012*, Medicine and Biomedical Sciences in Modern History,
https://doi.org/10.1007/978-3-030-18685-2_3

lines: class, gender and ethnicity, for instance, all figured in the way public health thought of and dealt with the public. Finally, the public was also conceived as a collection of individuals. The growing emphasis on individual behaviour in both causing and responding to public health problems helped to consolidate a focus on individuals and the risks they posed or encountered. Yet, these neat categories were rarely so well-defined in practice. Collective, group and individual ways of imagining the public often overlapped and sometimes conflicted with one another. Moreover, public health practitioners' conceptions of the public interacted with pre-existing assumptions and values. This resulted in a fractured, but dynamic, sense of the public. Public health actors' conception of the public, we argue, was multifaceted, sometimes contradictory, and open to change over time.

The chapter is divided into three sections. In the first, we examine how public health actors saw the public as an entirety. The epidemiological survey was an important tool for creating a sense of the population as a whole, as well as a collection of groups and individuals. Collective ways of viewing the public can also be seen in initiatives such as mass vaccination, where individuals were expected to undergo a procedure to benefit themselves and others. This mass public intersected with the new focus on individuals and their lifestyles, something observed in the 'invention' of exercise as a behaviour that was good for everybody. In Section Two, we get to grips with some of the ways the public were thought of as a collection of specific (albeit sometimes overlapping) groups. We examine how particular groups were made, used and applied by public health actors. Our focus is on class, gender and ethnicity. Other groups, were, of course, important, but these categories exorcised the most interest and also linked back to older ways of viewing and responding to the public. In Section Three, we reflect on how the public was imagined as a collection of individuals. Particularly important here is the emphasis on personal risk and individual behaviour, but this view of the public was not wholly atomised. Individuals were still often thought of as being part of particular groups, and some kinds of behaviour could be seen as a universal as well as an individual attribute. Throughout the chapter, we look at the imaginings of different types of public health actor, including government officials, public health researchers, health educators and medical practitioners. We conclude by reflecting on the three ways of viewing the public, and how these changed and stayed the same over time.

1 Public = Population

Despite the general move towards focusing on individual behaviour as a leading cause of ill-health over the course of the last half of the twentieth century, public health practitioners and policymakers continued to think of the public as a whole. The primary way in which this conceptualisation operated was in relation to the public as the population. 'Population' is a multifaceted concept, but a particular understanding of population was produced by epidemiological surveys in the post-war period. We also examine a key population-level public health intervention—mass vaccination—and how this helped create a sense of a public that was more than a collection of groups and individuals. The notion of the public as population could incorporate a focus on individual behaviours that were thought to be universally beneficial, and we look at this in relation to exercise and heart disease.

1.1 Epidemiological Surveys

The technological innovations of social surveys, medical statistics and epidemiology were integral to the development of twentieth-century public health and its scientific credibility (Porter 1996). Public health's expansion and interpretation of statistics played a vital role in determining how population health was viewed by policymakers and what actions should be taken to improve it (Szreter 2002a). But it also encouraged a new, more comprehensive conception of the public in public health. Through epidemiological surveys the whole population had the potential to become an object of and participant in research, and the public was reconfigured as a 'whole' made up of many 'parts', categories, and individuals (Crook 2016, 295).

As Alain Desrosières explains, in the late nineteenth century 'statistical summing elicited a more general viewpoint than that of the doctors who, seeing only patients … had a different perspective of public health issues' (Desrosières 2010, 170). Rather than examining the individual, this 'general viewpoint' focused 'attention and debate' on the economic and social environment 'as an explanatory factor in mortality'. While Desrosières suggests that such statistical work was concerned with 'the improvement of health and sanitary conditions in an urban environment', Seth Koven describes similar social surveys as a method of knowing 'the unknown slums' in cities expanding under industrial capitalism (Desrosières 2010, 169). Middle-class philanthropists and social reformers utilised the survey 'to know, to contain, to control, and to speak about the poor', often using terms of moral judgment (Koven 1991, 370). In the twentieth century, social scientists picked up the mantle conducting social surveys which focused on a public of unemployed or working people 'whose lives were impoverished and marginalised' over those who were 'prosperous and secure' (Lawrence 2013, 274–75).

The interest in those deemed to be 'impoverished and marginalised' was widely shared by researchers, social workers, the clergy, the police, doctors, and within public health. Public health practice largely focussed on women and children, sending sanitary inspectors and health visitors into communities to monitor and educate throughout the nineteenth and early twentieth centuries (Berridge 2007, 188; Davies 1988). In these accounts of social surveys, research was concerned with classifying populations, aiming to 'elicit, pathologize, and sometimes exoticize the morally deviant', separating them from the respectable and legitimate (Savage 2010, 7). Yet, as Desrosières asserts, in the early twentieth century, new sampling methods opened up a wider public to researchers. Rather than necessitating exhaustive surveys into poverty-stricken areas, representative sampling allowed parts to 'replace the whole', leading to a new conception of the 'whole' (Desrosières 2010, 226).

By the 1940s, social medicine was emphasising the dynamic relationship between health and social factors, aiming to explore how social and economic change affected health. Furthermore, practitioners refused to view health and sickness as absolute states and instead used statistical methods to examine 'norms and ranges of variation with respect to individual differences'; bringing this new 'whole' public under the purview of public health (Murphy and Smith 1997, 3). As a discipline, social medicine focused on building statistical links between 'life hazards, poor environments and poor health' and conceived of medicine as a social science which examined the social relations of health and to rectify inequalities (Oakley and Barker 2004, 5–6). Debates around social medicine intersected with those around the planning of the NHS, drawing the suspicion of clinicians and doctors 'for questioning their focus on the individual patient at the expense of the wider public good' and for looking beyond their professional expertise to the field of medical statistics (Oakley and Barker 2004; Porter 2002). Social medicine as a political project identified whole population health as a social problem and looked to social science and epidemiological surveys to inform health policy.

The expanded focus of social medicine brought new members of the public to the attention of public health. Epidemiological surveys asked members of this new public about their material conditions and social status as well as their health, and certain sections of the public found themselves the subjects of social investigation for the first time. These people may have been familiar with survey methods intellectually but not with how it felt to be subjected to them. Publics made up of the middle classes and men, rather than the usual survey subjects of women and the marginalised poor, were placed under the lens of the Survey, and these newer publics did not always behave as the surveyed should. Consisting of people with greater social, economic and political capital, these publics could more easily speak back to public health. Positioning themselves as the 'subject[s] of rights' as well as of research, they called into question top-down narratives of expertise and the authority of state representatives (Crook 2016, 295). Although epidemiological studies viewed the public through the lens of population health, in practice they were still dealing with individual members of the public.

1.2 Mass Vaccination and Herd Immunity

Additional tensions between the notion of 'population' and the individuals that were its constituents can be observed in one of the key population-level public health interventions of the post-war era: mass vaccination. During the nineteenth century, vaccination against smallpox prompted considerable public opposition. Rooted in religious, scientific and class-based hostility, anti-vaccination campaigns highlighted conflict between the rights of individuals and the collective good (Durbach 2005). Although vaccination was, for most of the post-war period, less contentious than it had been in the nineteenth century, mass vaccination programmes still required negotiation between individuals and the wider public of which they were part (Blume 2017). Immunisation programmes exemplified collective risk for collective reward. The actual risk of complications arising from vaccination was slight. But this was not the only price paid by the public. Children were expected to endure the discomfort of the procedure. Parents of young children bore the inconvenience of presenting their children for vaccination and the difficulty of seeing their child in pain and dealing with any rashes or irritability that might follow. Large bureaucratic systems for procuring, distributing and administering vaccines to those who needed them took significant resources to fund and staff. And the long-standing relationship between pharmaceutical companies, research institutions and public funding bodies meant that the British public sector invested, and continues to invest, to protect individuals from communicable diseases (Blume 2017; Heller 2008).

The benefits of mass vaccination were, similarly, collective. The concept of herd immunity held that the more people immunised, the lower the possibility of other people becoming infected by a particular disease. This both worked as a form of epidemic prevention and as a benefit to those individuals who, for whatever reason, were not immunised. The most obvious benefits were those of cost reduction. The modest expense on vaccination systems was more than repaid by lower hospital admissions, reduced incapacity for work, disability and death. Such arguments became explicit from the 1970s, when the welfare state sought to deal with financial crises by investing in preventative care. But there are also cultural reasons for such an investment. As vaccination became a proven and widespread tool for preventing disease, publics themselves demanded protection in the form of vaccination. Thus, in the 1950s, when the American Jonas Salk announced the successful field trials of his vaccine against polio, the British government rushed through a vaccination programme to meet the demand from British citizens (Lindner and Blume 2006; Millward 2017). As Jacob Heller has argued, vaccination became a symbol of a modern, functioning Western nation—something that advanced countries had and backward states did not (Heller 2008). Moreover, as citizens came to expect that their governments would manage risks to their personal safety, they demanded that not only the government provide vaccination services, but that fellow citizens adhere to national guidelines and vaccinate their children for the good of the collective. Population-level measures like vaccination, therefore, did more than protect the masses: they also helped to underline the continued importance of the public as a whole to collective health, and to the actors in charge of it.

1.3 *Universalising Individual Behaviour: Exercise*

Such universal imaginings of the public were also interwoven with understandings of the impact of individual behaviour on health. One such example is the way in which exercise came to be understood as a behaviour that would benefit everyone, no matter their individual status or what group or groups they belonged to. In September 2009, shortly before his death, the *Financial Times* ran a weekend magazine feature on British epidemiologist Professor Jeremiah 'Jerry' Morris, headlined 'The man who invented exercise' (Kuper 2009). Two months later, his obituarists echoed this appraisal. Berridge, writing in *The Guardian*, asserted that Morris 'was the first researcher to demonstrate the connection between exercise and health' (Berridge 2009). This reputation was largely predicated on the research he conducted with the Social Medicine Research Unit (SMRU), and in particular the London Transport Workers study. This study established a link between physical activity and coronary heart disease (CHD) by noting the lower rates of morbidity and mortality among bus conductors compared to their more sedentary bus driver colleagues (Morris et al. 1953a, b). Through this research, and later studies of leisure-time activity among British civil servants, the SMRU developed a concept of exercise as a self-consciously modern response to a modern epidemic apparently born out of shifts in the post-industrial labour market. In 1961, at a symposium at Yale, Morris claimed that '[r]eduction of physical activity is surely one of the characteristic social changes of the present century, and automation promises to finish the job' (Morris 1961).

Morris's concerns were borne out empirically. Economic historian Andrew Newell characterised the structural changes in the British labour market over the twentieth century as being driven by the 'engine' of 'technological process, which completely transformed the occupations, industries, hours of work, and, most of all, the standard of living of British workers' (Newell 2007, 35). The results of this were clear. While in 1951 48.5% of workers were employed in manual jobs, this had declined to 38.5% by 1977. Over the same period, employment in managerial, professional and technical occupations (sedentary desk work) had increased from 8.2 to 26.7% (Newell 2007, 39).

The SMRU established a large longitudinal cohort study of mostly sedentary, desk-bound civil servants to investigate the potential links between leisure-time physical activity and CHD, finding that 'vigorous exercise' had a protective effect (Morris et al. 1973). This, rather than the earlier London Transport Workers Study, was the point at which exercise, as the twenty-first-century headline writers of the *Financial Times* might have understood it, was invented. Exercise was defined, not as a quotidian by-product of an active and physically strenuous job, but as a set of leisure-time activities that have to be consciously performed to a certain level of vigour to compensate for one's sedentary day job. As Morris explained: 'Vigorous exercise is very different from just a general increase in physical activity, and a clear message is needed as to which forms of exercise are most beneficial' (Morris et al. 1973, 222).

The wider cultural influence of the SMRU research is necessarily diffuse and difficult to trace alongside other developments in post-industrial consumer societies, but as Dorothy Porter has argued, '[c]ommercialized physical culture expanded slowly after the Second World War up to the late 1970s and then made an exponential leap' (Porter 2011, 77). Exercise, at least in the SMRU and Morris's conception, was reinvented as a response to a modern epidemic (CHD), a result of modern sedentary lifestyles brought about by a modern macroeconomic shift (an increase in desk-bound work). The interwar construction of exercise as the action of responsible citizens in pursuit of the national health had been reconstituted.

Physical activity in post-war Britain was still very much part of the practice of citizenship, but now as an individualised, scientifically rational, modern way of life (Grant 2016). Alongside eating healthily and not smoking, exercise was a central tenet of public health's new focus on lifestyle. This was illustrated by policy documents such as the UK government's 1976 discussion paper *Prevention and Health: Everybody's Business*, which framed individuals' preventive health practices as a *quid pro quo* for the continuation of a health service free at the point of use as the NHS struggled financially (Department of Health and Social Security 1976). Further examples of exercise as literally 'active' citizenship were evident in the 1980s health promotion campaign 'Look After Your Heart' (memorably fronted by junior health minister Edwina Currie on an exercise bike), and the series of guidelines on physical activity published by the Chief Medical Officer, most recently in 2010 (Bull 2010). An individual behaviour could thus be a universal requirement for the entire population.

2 The Public = Groups

While 'the public' could be seen as being synonymous with the citizenry, or the whole population, this mass public was often sub-divided into smaller groups. The composition of these groups was determined by various factors. Socio-economic status (class) had long been a way of grouping supposedly similar people together, as had gender and ethnicity. In the post-war period, the make-up and nature of such groups were both consolidated and complicated by the rise of identity politics. The growth of new social movements helped to create new ways of identifying people, and new ways for people to identify themselves. Moreover, identities could be multiple: a gay man could also belong to an ethnic minority group and to the working-class. In this section, we do not aim to deal with every kind of identity group or with multiple identities. Rather, we focus on class, gender and ethnicity as three key groupings deployed by public health policymakers and practitioners. We highlight similarities and differences across these groups, and with past ways of imagining the public.

2.1 *Class*

The notion of 'class' is a mutable and disputed concept, and as a result the use of class in the context of public health in post-war Britain was always heterogeneous. Furthermore, as Mike Savage points out, class and class identities underwent considerable change over the course of the second half of the twentieth century (Savage 2008, 2010). Class was (and remains) a slippery, but profoundly important, category for public health actors and the ways they thought about and responded to the public. Writing in the 1970s, the Marxist theorist Raymond Williams discussed class extensively in *Keywords*, his 'vocabulary of culture and society'; tracing the brief history of the term, and what it meant in the present day. As a prominent public intellectual who was influential in contemporary discussions about cultural phenomena, his definition provides a useful lens with which to view class in public health, both contextually and theoretically. For Williams, three 'variable meanings of class' were used 'in a whole range of contemporary discussion and controversy … usually without clear distinction'. Class could mean either a 'group' (a socio-economic category), a 'rank' (indicating relative social position) or lastly 'formation', to describe organisation along social, political or cultural boundaries (Williams 1973, 66). All three meanings were mobilised at different points, and by various actors in British public health, throughout the second half of the twentieth century. In this section, we examine the ways in which class as both 'group' and 'rank' was instrumentalised by public health practitioners and policymakers. In Sect. 3, we consider how 'formation' mapped on to understandings of individual behaviour not only in relation to class, but to other identity categories too.

Of Williams's three meanings of class, 'group', or the '(objective) social or economic category' of class can be best observed in the design and delivery of public health surveys (Williams 1973, 66). Generally, public health surveys focused on this understanding of class by categorising the public into different class 'groups', by asking questions about income and about occupation and examining the material status of respondents. In 1911, the

Registrar General introduced a 'five-part social class stratification' which was soon adopted by other social investigators and went on to 'dominate demographic work during the twentieth century' (Webster 2002, 83; Renwick 2016, 14). Simon Szretzer has termed this the 'professional model of social classes' (Szreter 2002b). Chris Renwick notes that the 'professional model' marked a 'significant departure from earlier approaches to social structure because it identified status with work – that is, occupation – rather than worth'.

The Government Social Survey (GSS) department's Survey of Sickness, which ran from 1943 until 1952, followed this five-part model. The instructions given to interviewers working on the Survey described the 'economic classification' of subjects as follows; 'this is a broad grouping on an occupational basis, designed to show whether people who are on a level economically have similar characteristics in other respects, and whether different levels have different problems and needs in relation to a particular inquiry … The coding should be made on the basis of the occupation of the chief wage-earner, assisted, where possible, by knowing his/her wage rate' (Survey of Sickness Instructions to Interviewers 1945, 17). Although the Survey did ask about income, this was secondary to occupation: 'The occupation is of great importance and every effort should be made to obtain it precisely' (Survey of Sickness Instructions to Interviewers). Wage-rates and occupations were stratified together with occupations such as 'pensioners' and 'women in a variety of unskilled jobs' making up the bottom rung of 'Up to £3. 0. 0. a week', and, at the other end of the scale, male 'Managers', 'Management', 'Managerial staff' and 'Heads of Department' working in various trades filled the 'Over £10. 0. 0. a week' highest earning category (Survey of Sickness Instructions to Interviewers 1945, 17–20).

Although relatively straightforward, these classifications were not without controversy. In 1945, redrafted instructions to interviewers noted that the 'difficulty most widely experienced … is that of asking the Income Group of the Chief Wage Earner' (Survey of Sickness Instructions to Interviewers). Even those who understood the necessity of putting health in a social context, sometimes expressed annoyance with having to reveal their income in person and on the doorstep (Complaints Received from Members of the Public Interviewed by S.S. Investigators). A common grievance, it was discussed in detail by survey staff. The GSS issued each fieldworker with a card printed with income categories so that the survey subject could 'indicate … his income' non-verbally (Survey of Sickness Instructions to Interviewers 1945). Such difficulties were not unique to the 1940s and

1950s. In 2010, a report from the Health Survey for England found that there was some reluctance to answer newly included questions on contraception and sexual health, but 'item non-response was no higher than to other sensitive questions such as that on household income' (Robinson et al. 2011, 5).

Depending on the purpose of the study, health surveys sometimes tried other ways of categorising class. In the late 1950s, influenced by notions of class explored in Wilmott and Young's *Family and Kinship in East London*, Stephen Taylor and Sidney Chave asked respondents to their study of mental health in Harlow to self-define their social class alongside the by now-standard occupation and income questions (Young and Wilmott 2013). It did not go well. Half-way through the fieldwork, Chave wrote in his diary, 'I have decided to drop the Social Class Question from the interview. Several times the interviewers have said they feel awkward about putting this question: it has sometimes aroused the emotions of informants who say they don't believe in classes… one reluctant woman said to [an interviewer] – "I know you are going to ask me something silly about what social class I belong to"' (Facing the Winter). For the most part, throughout the post-war period public health surveys continued to use a combination of occupation and income to stratify class, although the specified wage-rates increased and occupations given as examples changed. Assigning individuals to particular socio-economic categories was important for public health researchers as it enabled them to track distinctions between and within groups. As historian Charles Webster noted, a British tradition of observing inequalities between social groups was nothing new: this goes at least as far back as Edwin Chadwick or Friedrich Engels (Webster 2002). Nevertheless, 'although inequalities in health have represented a continuing and serious social problem, active investigation tends to have been a periodic phenomenon, stimulated by perceptions of social crisis' (Webster 2002, 82). Historians such as Dorothy Porter have argued that in the immediate post-war years the 'pre-war political mission of social medicine to tackle health inequalities' was lost, with a 'shift of focus from social structure to social behaviour in the sociological analysis of disease and health' (D. Porter 2002, 70). In the late 1970s however—one of Webster's 'crisis' periods—there was a renewed focus on class and social inequality as a key determinant of health. This culminated in the August 1980 publication of the Black Report, a document widely viewed by both historians and public health campaigners as a pivotal moment in bringing the neologism of 'health inequalities' to public attention (Berridge 2002). The Black Report proved to be the catalyst for a decade's worth of activity on health inequalities by a loose network of epidemiologists, sociologists and campaigners. This focus on class as a key analytical prism through which public health viewed its public was maintained into the 1990s, with Donald Acheson's report on health inequalities in 1998, and the following decade with the Marmot Review, published in 2010 (Acheson 1998; Marmot 2010).

It is ironic, then, that one of the most influential analyses of health inequalities, the two Whitehall studies of London civil servants, started in 1968 with little or no thought given to investigating such issues. A relatively conventional risk factor study in the mould of the famous American-based Framingham project, the first Whitehall study recorded the grades of the male participants apparently merely as a 'matter of good housekeeping' (Marmot 2002; Oppenheimer 2005). According to the directors of the second Whitehall study, this followed the epidemiological conventions of the day:

> "social class" was not an object of study but a control variable: a potential confounder that you got rid of in order to arrive at the "correct" conclusion about the association between risk factor and disease. (Marmot and Brunner 2005)

As the study progressed however, startling inequalities became apparent; '[m]en in the lowest grade (messengers) had 3.6 times the [coronary heart disease] mortality of men in the highest employment grade (administrators)', a trend that was proportionately observed across all grades (Marmot and Brunner 2005). What contributed most significantly to this disparity? Was it their socio-economic status (i.e. 'group'); the behaviours that made up their 'formation' as a grade or social class; or was it their 'rank', their place in the hierarchy?

Ultimately, the Whitehall researchers decided that the latter explanation was most compelling. In a 1981 paper, they excluded absolute poverty as having anything to do with heart disease: '[e]xperience in Third World countries shows that where poverty is prevalent, coronary heart disease is rare'. The researchers also discounted many of the lifestyle risk factors, concluding that 'a man's employment status was a stronger predictor of his risk of dying from coronary heart disease than any of the more familiar risk factors' (Rose and Marmot 1981, 17). Only a third of the disparities in deaths from heart disease between grades could be explained by known risk factors such as cholesterol, obesity, smoking or sedentary lifestyles (Marmot and

Elliott 2005, 6). For the Whitehall researchers, 'rank' was the most powerful way of viewing the effects of class on health. They strongly argued that their findings were neither particular to civil servants nor Britain. Indeed, they even supplemented their findings with those of neurobiologist Robert Sapolsky in his studies of baboons and their own social orders. Whitehall II director Michael Marmot argued that inequalities in health had been found across Western nations, even those that thought they were relatively egalitarian, such as Sweden. As he noted, 'Whitehall, far from representing an atypical postimperial backwater, [was] typical of the developed world' (Marmot 2006, 1304). Class was thus profoundly important to the way public health actors imagined the public, but also to the health problems that members of the public were thought to encounter.

2.2 Gender

Socio-economic status was not the only method by which public health practitioners and policymakers categorised the public. From at least the nineteenth century onwards, there were gender divisions in imaginings of the public. Women were often the target of key public health initiatives such as the improvement of child health and hygiene in the home. In the post-war era, women, especially in their role as wives and mothers, continued to be a key focus for public health work. For instance, gendered assumptions about family life were integral to the way population health surveys were organised in the post-war period. The positioning of women as wives was fundamental to the structure of surveys and influenced the ways women responded to them and the information that they gathered. This can be seen in the GSS's Survey of Sickness which ran from 1943 until 1952. This was a study to measure the incidence of illness and injury in the whole population of England and Wales. Throughout its run, Government fieldworkers interviewed a representative sample of around 300,000 people about their health (Taylor 1958). In its instructions to interviewers written in 1945, the GSS defined 'any woman who is mainly responsible for the domestic duties of the household' as a 'housewife' whether she worked outside the home or not (Survey of Sickness Instructions to Interviewers 1945). Although 'housewife' was described as a form of 'other occupation', the survey was also clear that 'housewife' was a relationship. When categorising every individual they interviewed, the interviewers were instructed to: 'Please be careful to give relationship to the housewife and not to any other person' (Survey of Sickness Instructions to Interviewers

1945, 16). The questionnaire schedule was designed on the assumption that there would be a 'housewife' in the household and that she played a crucial role in household life. Questions about the house—the number of habitable rooms for example—were to be answered by the 'housewife' if she was present and the 'chief wage earner' only if she was not. It was suggested that 'in the few households' without a 'housewife', the 'relationship of different members to one another' should be made 'clear in a note' and attached (Survey of Sickness Instructions to Interviewers 1945). The organisation of the survey thus privileged the role of women in the home and conferred responsibility for knowledge about health and the home onto women, even when they were not the subjects of surveys themselves.

One result of this was that women, particularly wives, were often used as proxies in the absence of their husbands. The instructions to interviewers working on the Survey of Sickness asserted that 'in general a man is not a good proxy for a woman', but specifically mentioned that women; wives, daughters and mothers, could be used as proxies for men (Survey of Sickness Instructions to Interviewers 1945, 6). Many social researchers expected women to be knowledgeable about 'stomachs, homes and emotions' and to be willing to report on them (Anatomy of Don't Knows 1947). As Caitriona Beaumont and Amy Whipple have shown, the gendered assumption of household knowledge was widespread during the 1950s and early 1960s, and was often utilised by middle-class women's organisations to enact active forms of citizenship (Whipple 2010, 334). Groups such as the Mothers' Union, Women's Institute and Townswomen's Guilds responded enthusiastically to government requests for their views in order to place the voices of housewives 'right at the heart' of post-war reconstruction (Beaumont 2015, 146). In trusting women to act as proxies for members of their households, the GSS recognised this form of expertise. But this recognition was not always experienced by the women's husbands, some of whom wrote to complain. One irate man demanded in 1947: 'What authority have you to question my wife … regarding my personal health?' (Complaints Received from Members of the Public Interviewed by S.S. Investigators 1947). Claire Langhamer suggests that men and women experienced different meanings of home in the 1950s, and developed different understandings of domestic privacy (Langhamer 2005, 344). When considered alongside Kate Fisher's work which indicates that communication about sensitive issues between spouses was not always frequent or detailed, this puts the use of proxies into perspective (Fisher 2008). The health surveys' privileging of women's roles within the home led them to trust women's knowledge of their husbands' health more than the men in question did. Although the emphasis on women as 'housewives' has somewhat disappeared over the decades as labour practices altered and more women work outside the home, population-wide health surveying has continued to centre on households, focussing on the family unit.

Viewed as the primary caregivers to children, mothers were often the point of contact for health authorities seeking to monitor and intervene in the health of children. For infants and young children, this could be facilitated by home visits and mothers bringing their children to infant welfare clinics. For older children, the School Medical Service could deal more directly with pupils, albeit with the expressed written permission of the parents—most often assumed to be the mother (Daly 1983; Davis 2012). One place where mothers figured significantly was in attempts to increase childhood vaccination rates. When there were difficulties in vaccination campaigns, mothers were often positioned as the cause of problems and the targets for solutions. At the population level, mothers could be accused of apathy. When the diphtheria immunisation rate among infants dropped significantly in 1949/1950, health authorities blamed mothers for not fearing the disease. Advertising campaigns in particularly poorly performing districts stressed the need for immunisation and focused on the relationship between mother and baby. In specific instances, accusations could be even more direct and moralising. A series of outbreaks of diphtheria in Coseley, Staffordshire, led to scathing attacks on mothers' lack of care from local and national authorities (Ministry of Health 1954, 3, 34).

Despite such 'apathy', immunisation was increasingly seen as a common part of 'good' childrearing in the modern welfare state. The narrative around vaccinating children played on dominant notions of parenthood—which, in turn, often focused on motherhood. In the 1950s, literature and advertising made frequent references to 'parents' in gender-neutral terms, and fathers were not absent from discussions about vaccination, as shown through responses to government surveys on why children had or had not been immunised (Box 1945; Gray and Cartwright 1951). However, the dominance of the mother figure when discussing public health measures for children cannot be ignored. In the anti-poliomyelitis campaigns of the 1950s, for example, mothers' attitudes were the main target of Ministry of Health advertising (Anti-Poliomyelitis Vaccination Publicity to Raise Acceptance Rate 1959). Later, mothers would take on a dual role as both guardians to young children in need of vaccination and, as the programme expanded to young adults and expectant mothers, recipients of vaccination themselves. Even in the twenty-first century, the mother remains central to vaccination policy and practice. Regular surveys of parental attitudes to childhood immunisation question mothers rather than fathers, since women remain the most influential in decision making on a child's vaccination status (Yarwood et al. 2005).

The role of women in vaccination was not, however, confined to decisions about their own child's immunisation status. Women also actively took part in spreading public health messages, such as through the leafletting campaigns instigated by the Women's Institute for smallpox vaccination (Correspondence between Ministry of Health and Women's Voluntary Service and Women's Institute). Indeed, mothers' activism became increasingly important for government policy as the century progressed. While women's groups could help in education efforts, they could also resist and complicate vaccination programmes. Both the Association of Parents of Vaccine Damaged Children (1974) and Justice Awareness and Basic Support (1995) were founded by mothers who claimed their children had been damaged by vaccines (Fox 2006; JABS 2001). As vaccination crises grew around the contested safety of the whooping cough vaccine in the 1970s, and the measles-mumps-rubella vaccine in the 1990s, such groups were often able to use the media to promote their messages and demand compensation and policy changes from the governments of the day. This would suggest that mothers were not just the targets of public health initiatives but also active participants. Gendered views of the public mattered not only to public health officials, but to the public itself.

2.3 Ethnicity

Over the course of the second half of the twentieth century, ethnicity came to figure more centrally in the ways public health practitioners imagined the public. Race-based understandings of health and disease had long been present in Britain, but ethnicity as a distinct, identifiable category that could be linked to particular public health patterns and problems attracted little attention until the 1960s. This is evident in how ethnicity figured (or did not) in public health surveys. In the immediate post-war period, public health surveys ignored ethnicity. There were no questions regarding ethnicity in prominent public health surveys such as the GSS's Survey of Sickness (1943–1952) or the National Survey of Health and Development's 1946 Birth Cohort Study. Surveys collected information about income and occupation, to explore class, sex and age, but did not categorise the public in terms of ethnicity or 'race'.

The reasons for this are complex. First, the absence of an ethnicity question on many health surveys suggests that public health in the 1940s and 1950s often imagined the British public as white. In 1951, the black and minority ethnic (BME) population of Britain was estimated at around 74,500 (Waters 1997, 209). Although this rose throughout the 1950s to 336,000 by the end of 1959, and reached close to half a million people by the time the Commonwealth Immigrants Act came into effect in 1962, Chris Waters has suggested that 'Britishness and whiteness became increasingly synonymous' in the 1950s, partly through the 'exclusion of a racial other' (Waters 1997, 212). Another possible reason for the absence of questions regarding ethnicity in the 1940s and 1950s was the impact of the Second World War and the Holocaust on scientific thinking about 'race' (Barkan 1993; Stepan 1982). The Pearsonian statistics used in public health had developed alongside theories of eugenics and 'racial' science, or scientific racism (Renwick 2016; Schaffer 2008; Higgs 2000; Magnello 2002). Although some have downplayed the influence of eugenicist thought on medical statisticians, there was a clear link between eugenic ideas and population statistics, including those of population health (Magnello 2002). During the Second World War, scientists in Britain and internationally began to distance themselves from Nazism and the ideas of 'racial' science. After the war, scientists and social scientists from all over the world rejected biological understandings of race, as evidenced by the 1950 and 1952 UNESCO statements on 'race' (Schaffer 2007). These two statements argued that 'for all practical social purposes "race" is not so much a biological phenomenon as a social myth … given similar degrees of cultural opportunity to realize their potentialities, the average achievement of the members of each ethnic group is about the same' (Schaffer 2007, 260). With this in mind, questions regarding ethnicity, nationality or even 'race' may have been purposefully left out of population health surveys.

Such issues, however, could not be ignored for long. Waters has argued that the growing numbers of people of colour settling in Britain in the 1950s led to 'the emergence of a new "science," that of "race relations," pioneered by anthropologists and sociologists' who set out to 'study migrant communities and the response to them in Britain' and the differences in opportunity afforded to members of different ethnic groups (Waters 1997). At the same time, discussions around 'race' and discrimination became part of the agenda of mainstream politics. In the wake of the Notting Hill riots of 1958, the Labour Party 'issued a statement on "Racial Discrimination", committing a future Labour government to anti-discrimination legislation' (Schaffer 2014, 253). While public health authorities concerned themselves with the 'classic "port health" diseases' of tuberculosis and smallpox in relation to migration, public health surveys were slower to turn their focus onto migrant communities, never mind British-born people of colour (Bivins 2015, 14–15). In 1960, public health researcher Sidney Chave expressed surprise that his random sample of households in Harlow had selected a German family and an Indian family. Chave described them as an 'unusual batch of families', but this remark was the extent of his interest despite the Harlow mental health study's focus on migration to new towns (The End of Fieldwork 1960). Chave's survey did not ask questions about ethnicity. Although question 11 of the survey had asked 'Where do you come from?', which was suggestive of 'birthplace' questions in later surveys, the phrasing of question 12, 'How long had you lived in that district?', indicated that the expected answer was another town or county rather than country or continent (Taylor and Chave 1964, 209–10).

In the 1960s, when public health surveys began to address ethnicity directly, they did so in a way that embodied the tensions of the race relations project. As Waters notes, 'race relations experts consistently narrated the migrant other as a "stranger" to assumed norms of what it meant to be British' (Waters 1997, 209). Public health surveys dealt with ethnicity through the lens of migration. In 1958, the National Child Development Study Birth Cohort did not ask its participant mothers for their ethnicity. However, in 1965, the year of the first Race Relations Act, when the Study conducted their first follow up interviews, 'immigrants born in the reference week' were added into the sample (Power and Elliott 2006, 34). Ethnicity continued to be elided with the place of birth into the 1970s, but there were other, more biological understandings of ethnicity at work too. In 1971, the Office of Population Censuses and Surveys (OPCS) Social Survey Division began their General Household Survey (GHS), the health section of which picked up where the GSS Survey of Sickness had left off (Moss 1991, 159). The GHS asked questions about the ethnicity of respondents, including it as a category of analysis alongside class and sex. Respondents were asked for their parents' country of birth and interviewers were asked 'to code as "coloured" all those people who are not, in their estimation, "white"' (Office of Population Censuses and Surveys: Social Survey Division 1973, 75). The interviewers' instructions clarified that this meant 'Negros, brown skinned people such as Indians and Pakistanis, and yellow skinned people such as Chinese and Japanese' (Office of Population Censuses and Surveys: Social Survey Division 1973, A63). The GHS report indicated that the 'colour classification that results is not claimed to be either scientific or objective; however, it is expected to be reasonably consistent, meaningful and reproducible' (Office of Population Censuses and Surveys: Social Survey Division 1973, 75). The birthplace question operated on the understanding that the majority of BME people living in Britain were either first or second generation 'immigrants', with the 'colour' question acting as a way to discern 'white people … included among those whose parents had been born in the Indian subcontinent' and 'people whose parents were born in East Africa [but] were in fact of Asian descent' (Sillitoe and White 1992, 142). In 1975, the OPCS began to devise and trial questions on ethnicity which would provide more reliable information than parent's birthplace in recognition of the growing British-born BME population, but which were ultimately rejected by both the public and the Government before the 1981 Census (Sillitoe and White 1992, 144, 147).

The inclusion and exclusion of ethnicity from public health surveys in post-war Britain shows the malleable nature of the public and how conceptions of the public changed to fit the politics of the time. Like class and gender, dominant ideas about ethnicity were at work when public health practitioners imagined the public. These conceptions, however, took on distinct forms as they interacted with formulations that were specific to public health, such as the growing importance assigned to individual behaviour as both cause and cure for many public health problems.

3 Public = Individual Behaviours

As well as being seen as specific groups, the public could be broken down into even smaller units: that of individuals. Although this might seem somewhat contradictory, as 'the public' is often seen as referring to the masses, or at least large groups, in the context of public health there was a special impetus towards imagining the public as a set of individuals.

From the 1950s onwards, epidemiologists and others began to establish links between individual behaviour and diseases such as certain types of cancer and heart disease. This meant that public health practitioners and policymakers had to take greater interest in individuals and their actions. In this section, we discuss some of the ways in which this focus on individuals was manifested within post-war public health, especially in connection with ideas about risk and the communication of this through health education. We contend that ways of thinking about individuals often aligned with ways of thinking about groups. Class, gender and ethnicity once more came to the fore. At the same time, there was also a countervailing tendency to think about some of the more universal aspects of individual behaviour, as something that the entire public, no matter which group they belonged to, needed to take into account.

3.1 Risk

One of the most important means by which individual behaviour came to be seen as a causal factor in disease aetiology was through the development of the notion of 'risk'. The linking of chronic disease to lifestyle relied upon a statistical understanding of certain behaviours or characteristics and the likelihood that these would lead to ill-health. Beginning in America in the late 1950s and early 1960s, but spreading rapidly around the developed world, 'risk factors' for specific diseases were identified, such as high cholesterol and blood pressure for CHD (Rothstein 2003; Oppenheimer 2006; Timmermann 2012). Although risk factors were thought to be universal in their biological or behavioural nature, these were not evenly distributed across the population. Certain groups were thought to be more at risk than others due to their behaviour and characteristics.

This can be seen in relation to understandings of CHD. For much of the twentieth century, heart disease was conceived, by default, as a male disease. When CHD emerged as an apparent epidemic in Western nations in the immediate post-war period, its most visible, and most numerous, victims were middle-aged men (Ehrenreich 1984, 70–73). Large cohort studies in Britain that attempted to tease out the causes of the epidemic were conducted exclusively with male participants. The first Whitehall study, which started in 1968, only included male civil servants (Marmot and Brunner 2005, 251). Ten years later, the British Regional Heart Study recruited 7735 middle-aged men, and no women (Walker, Whincup, and Shaper 2004). An editorial in *The Lancet* in 1991 puzzled over these omissions, arguing that 'in most developed countries CHD is unquestionably the biggest killer in women as well as in men and a cause of considerable morbidity' and that 'there is no sex difference in the mechanism of CHD, so the classic risk factors should apply' (Anon. 1991).

This omission of women from research agendas was informed by cultural understandings of heart attacks as being the blight of the male breadwinner, intrinsically connected with work and stress. Studies of heart disease in the immediate post-war years were keen to investigate the links between occupation and heart disease, while the persistent popularity of the Type A hypothesis—that alpha males with highly ambitious personalities were more likely to be stressed and consequently suffer heart attacks—meant that even as the workforce became increasingly feminised, heart disease continued to be highly masculinised (Aronowitz 1988). Historian Jane Hand has illustrated such conceptions in popular discourse by her close reading of Flora margarine advertising, tracing a history of 'the visual representation of the at-risk male, widening out to all males and finally re-incorporating the female purchaser and consumer' (Hand 2017, 479, 493). Hand suggests that by the mid-1980s 'women themselves were increasingly being identified as at-risk from CHD', but it was not until 1999 that the British Women's Heart and Health Study was established as a 'sister' study of the British Regional Heart Study (Hand 2017, 493). The persistence of the male coronary 'candidate' in the public and medical imagination was underlined in 2018 by news stories reporting that women suffered worse clinical outcomes following heart attacks, with the study author commenting that there was a 'misconception amongst the general public and healthcare professionals about what heart attack patients are like … [t]ypically, when we think of a heart attack patient, we see a middle-aged man who is overweight, has diabetes and smokes' (Anon. 2018).

Distinctions in risk profiling were not just linked to gender. In his discussion of post-war chronic disease research in former British colonies, Martin Moore has posited that the new methodologies of risk-factor epidemiology, and its 'harnessing [of] the power of difference', had important implications for domestic public health. Moore persuasively argues that British biomedical researchers compared and contrasted the ethnic, cultural and environmental differences of such populations in order to gain insight into the aetiology and risk factors for conditions such as hypertension, diabetes and heart disease. These research subjects of Commonwealth countries 'provided an "other" for the British population' in the post-war years (Moore 2016). But it was also new migrant communities in Britain that began to capture researchers' interests. One area where this can be observed is in the response to smallpox outbreaks from the late 1940s to the early 1960s. After its eradication from Britain in the 1930s, smallpox became intimately associated with a foreign threat (Arnold 1993, 116–58). All British cases in the post-war period could be traced to specific instances of importation, usually a named individual arriving by air or by sea from South Asia. In the 1940s and 1950s, India and later Pakistan were often associated with smallpox, but this characterisation applied to the lands rather than the people per se. Indeed, when an Australian couple died of smallpox on the SS Mooltan in 1950, causing some secondary infections among the British population, the authorities blamed the husband's behaviour. He had visited a Bengal bazaar against the advice of the health authorities and, as was common for his compatriots at the time, he was unvaccinated because smallpox was so rare in Australasia (Morgan 1950). Similarly, a 1949 outbreak in Glasgow was attributed to a 'Lascar' seaman who recovered in a Scottish hospital. His race was less important than the ports he had passed through, and when he had recovered he was given a fond farewell from the locals (Anon. 1950a, b). The British population appeared to show no ill-will to such isolated incidents.

This situation changed as the practices of Indian and Pakistani migrants became more politicised in the 1960s. During the height of debates on the Commonwealth Immigration Bill (which sought to limit 'coloured' immigration) in 1961/1962 a series of small outbreaks of smallpox linked to air travellers led to widespread calls for more restrictions on who could enter the country and more rigorous medical checks at ports (Bivins 2008). This was not grounded in epidemiological research. Port controls had performed well for decades and smallpox was becoming less of a threat to Britain due to significant progress in the global eradication programme conducted by the World Health Organization (Dick 1962; Dixon 1962). These were politically rooted demands aimed at controlling the behaviour of foreigners and citizens travelling to contaminated lands. For while the British public appeared to demand vaccination of immigrants and emigrants—British subjects required vaccination before visiting many countries, both to protect the host country and to avoid the traveller bringing back a communicable disease—infant vaccination rates against smallpox in the domestic population remained well below 35% in most districts (Immunisation and Vaccination Statistics 1964). Certain diseases, then, could be seen as solely a problem for outsiders and for adequate border control rather than problems that required changes in behaviour or inconvenience for the 'native' population. A 'risky' group posed a threat, but this could be controlled.

Although recent immigrants were initially discussed in medical and political circles in terms of infectious disease, by the 1970s and 1980s, according to Moore, 'doctors could no longer ignore the presence of black and Asian populations in British chronic disease clinics, and clinicians organised prevalence surveys and research programmes with the aim of determining resource implications for the NHS' (Bivins 2015; Moore 2016, 403). While it was acknowledged that there might be genetic and biological determinants (or 'susceptibility') to racialised conditions such as 'Asian rickets' or type 2 diabetes, the means of addressing these issues were placed firmly in the cultural and social sphere, most particularly with regard to migrant communities' dietary habits. Bivins cites the discussions over fortifying chapatti flour with vitamin D as a means to address rickets in children of South Asian descent (Bivins 2015, 252–55). Similarly, higher rates of heart disease among Bangladeshi, Pakistani and Indian men led the Health Education Authority (HEA) to publish a manual for prevention in 1994 that this group's recommended fat intake be reduced to 30% of total energy intake, in contrast to the 33% for the rest of the nation (McKeigue and Sevak 1994). At the time of writing, the British Heart Foundation continues to produce cookbooks specifically for south Asian and African-Caribbean audiences (British Heart Foundation 2012, 2013). Over time, then, attention had shifted from seeing ethnic minorities as posing a risk to the white population (through smallpox) to focusing on the health risks thought to be encountered by ethnic minority individuals.

3.2 *Targeting: Health Education*

The different patterns of disease among groups and individuals has been used to justify the targeting of health education initiatives to reach those most at risk. But such efforts also reflected and reinforced other assumptions about these various imagined publics and their behaviours. This can be observed in the ways class, gender and ethnicity figured in health education campaigns throughout the post-war period. The notion of class on display in health education can be aligned with Williams's description of class as 'formation', as it tended to focus on the impact of the social, political and cultural boundaries of distinctions between classes, and especially the tastes and lifestyles of different class categories. The habits of the working classes had long been of interest to health educators, especially around issues such as hygiene and cleanliness (Crook 2016). In the post-war period, the focus on what Jerry Morris described as 'ways of living', or 'mass habits and social customs' intensified as these became more strongly linked to disease and ill-health (Morris 1955). Although these habits could be found throughout the population, the efforts of health educators tended to focus on the behaviours of lower socio-economic groups. This was, as the Cohen

Report on health education remarked in 1964, because of the supposed 'difficulty of reaching people in lower social classes who may often be the most in need of education in health matters but the least ready to accept it' (Central Health Services Council and Scottish Health Services Council 1964, 36). Such perceptions continued across the decades. In a document describing their 'Look After Your Heart' campaign from 1987 the HEA asserted that their efforts were 'aimed at everyone in England. However, the prevalence of CHD is greatest among certain groups (mainly socio-economic groups C2, D and E), who have also proved the hardest to reach effectively with health education messages' (Health Education Authority 1987, 10).

As the HEA document hinted, the strategy of focusing health education on the poorer groups in society, was, to some degree, justified by the pattern of disease and its relationship to socio-economic status. People in lower social classes experienced worse health, but the extent to which this was related to behaviour, rather than the environment or social structure, was much more debateable. This can be seen in the case of smoking. During the 1950s and early 1960s, rates of smoking were even across the social classes. Yet, during the 1970s, smoking began to decline among the higher socio-economic groups (Berridge 2007, 206). It could be suggested that this was because the more affluent groups in society took on board anti-smoking messages and acted accordingly (Britten 2007). On the other hand, more nuanced research pointed to the value of smoking in the lives of poorer people and their reduced incentives for giving up smoking in order to benefit long-term health (Lawlor et al. 2003; Graham 1987). Health education, then, may not have 'succeeded' or 'failed' in relation to class as formation: it simply missed its target.

Further evidence for this can be found in how class figured in specific health education campaigns. Many of the early anti-smoking messages appeared to have been aimed at all socio-economic groups, but by the mid-1960s there was a more concerted attempt to reach working-class young people (Berridge and Loughlin 2005). Moreover, some of these campaigns made explicit use of a wider set of social and cultural objects and activities to encourage young people to stop smoking. In the Ministry of Health's 'More money, more fun if you don't smoke' poster from 1966, a young man is surrounded by high-value consumer goods which would have been items of desire for many working-class youths. Drawing on such aspirational imagery, could, however, backfire. A poster produced for the Health Education Council's 1977–1979 alcohol education campaign conducted in the North East of England made use of a picture of a manicured female hand reaching for a bottle of vodka. Yet, this image did not resonate with the intended working-class audience, and the entire campaign was found to be too geared towards a 'middle-class view of life' (Budd et al. 1983). This suggests that the long-running tension between largely middle-class public health practitioners and policymakers, and more working-class audiences, persisted. Moreover, it also indicates that class continued to matter in a variety of ways in post-war public health, even as more traditional class-based identities broke down and other methods of identifying and categorising people came to the fore.

Indeed, health education campaigns were not just targeted at changing the behaviours of the working classes, but at other groups thought to be most in need, including women and ethnic minorities. To some extent, these efforts could be related to the idea that individuals in such groups were at a higher risk of developing particular conditions, but other tropes were at work too. Gendered views of women's role as mothers, for instance, underpinned anti-smoking campaigns during the 1970s. According to Berridge, smoking was regarded largely as a male habit until the late 1960s. From this time onwards, female smoking appeared to be on the increase, especially among younger women. Other research suggested that female smokers had smaller babies and that smoking might contribute towards foetal and neonatal deaths. Such evidence appeared to justify an anti-smoking campaign targeted specifically at pregnant women, which was launched in 1973. Yet, as Berridge argues, the roots of the campaign went beyond concerns about foetal health (Berridge 2007, 187–93). As discussed above, mothers had long been the target of public health campaigns. There were also specific reasons why pregnant women, and the health of the foetus, prompted particular concern at this time. The late 1960s and early 1970s saw the introduction of legal abortion and the development of the contraceptive pill, potentially giving women more control over their reproductive health than ever before. Interest in pregnant smokers was not, therefore, just about reducing the health risks of a specific group, but can be related to deeper, longer running issues surrounding reproduction and who had the power to control it.

Similarly, broader ideas about race and ethnicity also help explain some of the health education campaigns targeted at ethnic minorities. The persistence of rickets among the South Asian population in Britain was linked by public health policymakers to diet, culture and skin colour. Although there were debates about how to address the issue, including fortification of staple foods or exposing affected groups to more sunlight, health education was settled on as the way forward. The 'Stop Rickets' campaign of the 1970s and 1980s was, as Bivins points out, saturated with assumptions about the Asian community and the superiority of the 'British' way of life. Asians were encouraged to eat a diet more like that of the white community by posters that made use of 'oriental' motifs and depictions of 'Asian' people. Rickets was framed as a specifically 'Asian' problem, with the tacit (and sometimes more overt) message that 'traditional' culture and diet was to blame (Bivins 2015, 278–91). Yet, as contemporaries noted, rickets was not the most pressing public health issue facing British Asians. In their analysis of health education materials designed for ethnic minorities during the 1980s Bhopal and Donaldson found that these focused on pregnancy and infant care as well as the prevention of rickets. But, they suggested, this did not necessarily reflect the health education needs of ethnic minorities which included information about the biggest killer (heart disease) and how to access health services. Bhopal and Donaldson argued that 'Health education services should focus not only on those health problems where the ethnic minority group has an excess of a problem as compared to the host population, but also where there is no difference, or indeed, where there is a deficit' (Bhopal and Donaldson 1988, 139).

4 Conclusion

Despite the growing interest in individuals and their behaviour over the course of the post-war period, group and mass ways of imagining the public persisted. Indeed, it was sometimes hard to separate these different publics. Individual behaviour was often tied to membership of a particular group. The distinctions between groups certainly mattered, but there were numerous public health initiatives, like vaccination, where the whole public was the target. Numerical and statistical ways of imaging the public could simultaneously emphasise individual risk, encompass never-before surveyed groups (like middle-class men) and conceptualise the public at the population level. Health education efforts were often targeted at individuals who were members of specific groups but were sometimes designed to reach everybody. This indicates that the rise of identity politics, coupled with the linking of chronic disease to individual behaviour, did not mark the end of a mass public. Indeed, as we explore in Chapter 4, the public itself came to matter to public health policy in practice in new and unexpected ways through its ability to 'speak back' to public health.

Archival Material

Mass Observation at The Keep, SxMOA1/1/12/12/6, 15: Anatomy of the 'Don't Knows,' December 1947.

The National Archives, RG 26/26: Survey of Sickness—Instructions to Interviewers, 1945.

The National Archives, RG 40/134: Complaints Received from Members of the Public Interviewed by S.S. Investigators, 9 May 1951.

The National Archives, RG 40/133: Complaints Received from Members of the Public Interviewed by S.S. Investigators, 6 May 1947.

The National Archives, MH 55/2212: S. A. Heald to various local authorities, Anti-Poliomyelitis Vaccination Publicity to Raise Acceptance Rate 23 October 1959.

The National Archives, MH 55/902: Correspondence with the Ministry of Health involving the Women's Voluntary Service and Women's Institute.

The National Archives, MH 154/61: Immunisation and Vaccination Statistics as at 31 December 1964.

Wellcome Library, GC/178/A/2/6: Facing the Winter, 26 October–24 December 1959.

Wellcome Library, GC/178/A/2/8: The End of the Field Work, 13 April 1960.

Bibliography

Acheson, Donald. 1998. *Independent Inquiry into Inequalities in Health.* London: The Stationary Office.

Anon. 1950a. 'Epidemiology Section.' *British Medical Journal* 1 (4658): 914–15.

———. 1950b. 'Moosa Ali Says "Sorry About the Epidemic".' *Daily Mail*, 20 April.

———. 1991. 'Fair of Face and Sick at Heart.' *Lancet (London, England)* 338 (8779): 1366–67.

———. 2018. 'Heart Attack Care Dangerously Unequal for Women, Study Finds.' *BBC News* (blog), 8 January. https://www.bbc.co.uk/news/health-42590013.

Arnold, David. 1993. *Colonizing the Body: State Medicine and Epidemic Disease in Nineteenth-Century India.* Berkeley: University of California Press.

Aronowitz, Robert. 1988. 'The Rise and Fall of the Type A Hypothesis.' In *Making Sense of Illness: Science, Society and Disease*, 145–65. Cambridge: Cambridge University Press.

Barkan, Elazar. 1993. *The Retreat of Scientific Racism: Changing Concepts of Race in Britain and the United States Between the World Wars.* Reprint ed. Cambridge and New York: Cambridge University Press.

Beaumont, Caitríona. 2015. *Housewives and Citizens.* Manchester: Manchester University Press.

Berridge, Virginia. 2002. 'The Black Report and the Health Divide.' *Contemporary British History* 16 (3): 131–72.

———. 2007. *Marketing Health: Smoking and the Discourse of Public Health in Britain, 1945–2000.* Oxford: Oxford University Press.

———. 2009. 'Jerry Morris Obituary.' *The Guardian*, 3 December. http://www.theguardian.com/science/2009/dec/03/jerry-morris-obituary.

Berridge, Virginia, and Kelly Loughlin. 2005. 'Smoking and the New Health Education in Britain 1950s-1970s.' *American Journal of Public Health* 95 (6): 956–64.

Bhopal, R. S., and L. J. Donaldson. 1988. 'Health Education for Ethnic Minorities—Current Provision and Future Directions.' *Health Education Journal* 47 (4): 137–40.

Bivins, Roberta E. 2008. '"The People Have No More Love Left for the Commonwealth": Media, Migration and Identity in the 1961–62 British Smallpox Outbreak.' *Immigrants & Minorities* 25 (October): 263–89.

———. 2015. *Contagious Communities: Medicine, Migration, and the NHS in Post-war Britain.* Oxford: Oxford University Press.

Blume, Stuart S. 2017. *Immunization: How Vaccines Became Controversial.* S.l.: Reaktion Books.

Box, Kathleen. 1945. *Diphtheria Immunisation: An Inquiry Made by the Social Survey for the Ministry of Health.* London: The Social Survey.

British Heart Foundation. 2012. *Traditional Foods—Healthy Dishes.* London: British Heart Foundation.

———. 2013. *Taste of South Asia.* London: British Heart Foundation.

Britten, Nick. 2007. 'Poor People "Ignore" Health Campaigns.' *Daily Telegraph*, 23 June. https://www.telegraph.co.uk/news/uknews/1555427/Poor-people-ignore-health-campaigns.html.

Budd, J., P. Gray, and R. McCron. 1983. *The Tyne Tees Alcohol Education Campaign: An Evaluation.* London: Health Education Council.

Bull, F. C. 2010. *Physical Activity Guidelines in the U.K.: Review and Recommendations.* Loughborough: Loughborough University.

Central Health Services Council and Scottish Health Services Council. 1964. *Health Education.* London: HMSO.

Crook, Tom. 2016. *Governing Systems: Modernity and the Making of Public Health in England, 1830–1910.* Oakland, CA: University of California Press.

Daly, Ann. 1983. *Inventing Motherhood: The Consequences of an Ideal.* New York: Schocken.

Davies, Celia. 1988. 'The Health Visitor as Mother's Friend: A Woman's Place in Public Health, 1900–14.' *Social History of Medicine* 1 (1): 39–59.

Davis, Angela. 2012. *Modern Motherhood: Women and Family in England, 1945–2000.* Manchester: Manchester University Press.

Department of Health and Social Security. 1976. *Prevention and Health: Everybody's Business. A Reassessment of Public and Personal Health*. London: HMSO.

Desrosières, Alain. 2010. *The Politics of Large Numbers: A History of Statistical Reasoning*. Translated by Camille Naish. New ed. Cambridge, MA: Harvard University Press.

Dick, G. W. A. 1962. 'Prevention of Virus Diseases in the Community.' *British Medical Journal* 2 (5315): 1275–80.

Dixon, C. W. 1962. *Smallpox*. London: J&A Churchill.

Durbach, Nadja. 2005. *Bodily Matters: The Anti-vaccination Movement in England, 1853–1907*. Durham, NC: Duke University Press.

Ehrenreich, Barbara. 1984. *The Hearts of Men: American Dreams and the Flight from Commitment*. Reprint ed. Garden City, NY: Anchor Books.

Fisher, Kate. 2008. *Birth Control, Sex, and Marriage in Britain 1918–1960*. Oxford: Oxford University Press.

Fox, Rosemary. 2006. *Helen's Story*. London: John Blake.

Graham, Hilary. 1987. 'Women's Smoking and Family Health.' *Social Science & Medicine* 25 (1): 47–56.

Grant, Matthew. 2016. 'Historicizing Citizenship in Post-war Britain.' *The Historical Journal* 59 (4): 1187–206.

Gray, P. G., and Ann Cartwright. 1951. 'Diphtheria Immunisation in 1951: An Inquiry Carried Out in May 1951 for the Ministry of Health.' SS 176. London: The Social Survey.

Hand, Jane. 2017. 'Marketing Health Education: Advertising Margarine and Visualising Health in Britain from 1964–c.2000.' *Contemporary British History* 31 (4): 477–500.

Health Education Authority. 1987. *Look After Your Heart: A Campaign to Encourage Healthier Lifestyles in England*. London: Health Education Authority.

Heller, Jacob. 2008. *The Vaccine Narrative*. Nashville: Vanderbilt University Press.

Higgs, Edward. 2000. 'Medical Statistics, Patronage and the State: The Development of the MRC Statistical Unit, 1911–1948.' *Medical History* 44: 323–40.

JABS. 2001. 'JABS, "Fair Warning".' 25 October. http://web.archive.org/web/20011025144125, http://www.jabs.org.uk:80/jabsinformation.htm.

Koven, Seth. 1991. 'The Dangers of Castle Building—Surveying the Social Survey.' In *The Social Survey in Historical Perspective*, edited by Martin Bulmer, Kevin Bales, and Kathryn Kish Sklar, 368–76. Cambridge and New York: Cambridge University Press.

Kuper, Simon. 2009. 'The Man Who Invented Exercise.' *Financial Times*, 12 September. http://www.ft.com/cms/s/0/e6ff90ea-9da2-11de-9f4a-00144feabdc0.html.

Langhamer, Claire. 2005. 'The Meanings of Home in Postwar Britain.' *Journal of Contemporary History* 40 (2): 341–62.

Lawlor, Debbie A., Stephen Frankel, Mary Shaw, Shah Ebrahim, and George Davey Smith. 2003. 'Smoking and Ill Health: Does Lay Epidemiology Explain the Failure of Smoking Cessation Programs Among Deprived Populations?' *American Journal of Public Health* 93 (2): 266–70.

Lawrence, Jon. 2013. 'Class, "Affluence" and the Study of Everyday Life in Britain, c. 1930–64.' *Cultural and Social History* 10 (2): 273–99.

Lindner, Ulrike, and Stuart Blume. 2006. 'Vaccine Innovation and Adoption: Polio Vaccines in the UK, the Netherlands and West Germany, 1955–1965.' *Medical History* 50 (4): 425–46.

Magnello, Eileen. 2002. 'The Introduction of Mathematical Statistics into Medical Research: The Roles of Karl Pearson, Major Greenwood and Austin Bradford Hill.' In *The Road to Medical Statistics*, edited by Eileen Magnello and Anne Hardy, 95–123. Amsterdam: Rodopi.

Marmot, Michael. 2002. M. Marmot, Interview with H. Kreisler, Conversations with History. http://globetrotter.berkeley.edu/people2/Marmot/marmot-con3.html.

———. 2006. 'Status Syndrome: A Challenge to Medicine.' *Journal of the American Medical Association* 295 (11): 1304–7.

———. 2010. 'Fair Society Healthy Lives (The Marmot Review).' http://www.instituteofhealthequity.org/resources-reports/fair-society-healthy-lives-the-marmot-review.

Marmot, Michael, and Eric Brunner. 2005. 'Cohort Profile: The Whitehall II Study'. *International Journal of Epidemiology* 34 (2): 251–56.

Marmot, Michael, and Paul Elliott, eds. 2005. *Coronary Heart Disease Epidemiology: From Aetiology to Public Health.* 2nd ed. Oxford and New York: Oxford University Press.

McKeigue, P., and L. Sevak. 1994. *Coronary Heart Disease in South Asian Communities: A Manual for Health Promotion.* London: Health Education Authority.

Millward, Gareth. 2017. '"A Matter of Commonsense": The Coventry Poliomyelitis Epidemic 1957 and the British Public.' *Contemporary British History* 31 (3): 384–406.

Ministry of Health. 1954. *Report of the Ministry of Health for the Year Ended 31st December, 1953 Part II on the State of the Public Health.* Cmd. 9307. London: HMSO.

Moore, Martin D. 2016. 'Harnessing the Power of Difference: Colonialism and British Chronic Disease Research, 1940–1975.' *Social History of Medicine* 29 (2): 384–404.

Morgan, Montagu Travers. 1950. *Annual Report of the Medical Officer of Health to 31st December, 1949.* London: Port of London Health Authority.

Morris, J. N. 1955. 'Uses of Epidemiology.' *British Medical Journal* 2 (4936): 395–401.

———. 1961. 'Epidemiological Aspects of Ischaemic Heart Disease.' *The Yale Journal of Biology and Medicine* 34 (3–4): 359–69.

Morris, J. N., J. A. Heady, P. A. Raffle, C. G. Roberts, and J. W. Parks. 1953a. 'Coronary Heart-Disease and Physical Activity of Work.' *Lancet (London, England)* 265 (6795): 1053–57.

———. 1953b. 'Coronary Heart-Disease and Physical Activity of Work.' *Lancet (London, England)* 265 (6796): 1111–20.

Morris, J. N., S. P. W. Chave, C. Adam, C. Sirey, L. Epstein, and D. J. Sheehan. 1973. 'Vigorous Exercise in Leisure-Time and the Incidence of Coronary Heart Disease.' *The Lancet* 301 (7799): 333–39.

Moss, Louis. 1991. *The Government Social Survey: A History.* London: HMSO.

Murphy, S., and G. D. Smith. 1997. 'The British Journal of Social Medicine: What Was in a Name?' *Journal of Epidemiology and Community Health* 51 (1): 2–8.

Newell, Andrew. 2007. 'Structural Change.' In *Work and Pay in 20th Century Britain*, edited by Nicholas Crafts, Ian Gazeley, and Andrew Newell, 35–54. Oxford: Oxford University Press.

Oakley, Ann, and Jonathan Barker, eds. 2004. *Private Complaints and Public Health: Richard Titmuss on the National Health Service.* Bristol: Policy Press.

Office of Population Censuses and Surveys: Social Survey Division. 1973. *The General Household Survey: Introductory Report.* London: HMSO.

Oppenheimer, Gerald M. 2005. 'Becoming the Framingham Study 1947–1950.' *American Journal of Public Health* 95 (4): 602–10.

———. 2006. 'Profiling Risk: The Emergence of Coronary Heart Disease Epidemiology in the United States (1947–70).' *International Journal of Epidemiology* 35 (3): 720–30.

Porter, Dorothy. 2002. 'From Social Structure to Social Behaviour in Britain After the Second World War.' *Contemporary British History* 16 (3): 58–80.

———. 2011. *Health Citizenship: Essays in Social Medicine and Biomedical Politics.* Berkeley and Los Angeles, CA: University of California Press.

Porter, Theodore M. 1996. *Trust in Numbers: The Pursuit of Objectivity in Science and Public Life.* New ed. Princeton, NJ: Princeton University Press.

Power, Chris, and Jane Elliott. 2006. 'Cohort Profile: 1958 British Birth Cohort (National Child Development Study).' *International Journal of Epidemiology* 35 (1): 34–41.

Renwick, Chris. 2016. 'Eugenics, Population Research, and Social Mobility Studies in Early and Mid-Twentieth Century Britain.' *The Historical Journal* 59 (3): 845–67.

Robinson, Chloe, Anthony Nardone, Catherine Mercer, and Anne E. Johnson. 2011. *Health Survey for England 2010: Chapter Six—Sexual Health.* London: TSO.

Rose, G., and M. G. Marmot. 1981. 'Social Class and Coronary Heart Disease.' *British Heart Journal* 45 (1): 13–19.

Rothstein, William G. 2003. *Public Health and the Risk Factor: A History of an Uneven Medical Revolution*. Rochester, NY: University of Rochester Press.

Savage, Mike. 2008. 'Affluence and Social Change in the Making of Technocratic Middle-Class Identities: Britain, 1939–55.' *Contemporary British History* 22 (4): 457–76.

———. 2010. *Identities and Social Change in Britain Since 1940: The Politics of Method*. Oxford and New York, NY: Oxford University Press.

Schaffer, Gavin. 2007. '"'Scientific' Racism Again?": Reginald Gates, the Mankind Quarterly and the Question of "Race" in Science After the Second World War.' *Journal of American Studies* 41 (2): 253–78.

———. 2008. *Racial Science and British Society, 1930–62*. 2008 ed. Basingstoke and New York: AIAA.

———. 2014. 'Legislating Against Hatred: Meaning and Motive in Section Six of the Race Relations Act of 1965.' *Twentieth Century British History* 25 (2): 251–75.

Sillitoe, K., and P. H. White. 1992. 'Ethnic Group and the British Census: The Search for a Question.' *Journal of the Royal Statistical Society. Series A (Statistics in Society)* 155 (1): 141–63.

Stepan, Nancy. 1982. *The Idea of Race in Science: Great Britain, 1800–1960*. Houndmills, Hampshire: Palgrave Macmillan.

Szreter, Simon. 2002a. 'Rethinking McKeown: The Relationship Between Public Health and Social Change.' *American Journal of Public Health* 92 (5): 722–25.

———. 2002b. *Fertility, Class and Gender in Britain, 1860–1940*. Cambridge: Cambridge University Press.

Taylor, Stephen. 1958. 'The Survey of Sickness, 1943–52: Was Our Survey Really Necessary.' *The Lancet* 271 (7019): 521–523.

Taylor, Stephen, James Lake, and Sidney Chave. 1964. *Mental Health and Environment*. London: Longmans.

Timmermann, Carsten. 2012. 'Appropriating Risk Factors: The Reception of an American Approach to Chronic Disease in the Two German States, c. 1950–1990.' *Social History of Medicine* 25 (1): 157–74.

Walker, Mary, P. H. Whincup, and A. G. Shaper. 2004. 'The British Regional Heart Study 1975–2004.' *International Journal of Epidemiology* 33 (6): 1185–92.

Waters, Chris. 1997. '"Dark Strangers" in Our Midst: Discourses of Race and Nation in Britain, 1947–1963.' *Journal of British Studies* 36 (2): 207–38.

Webster, Charles. 2002. 'Investigating Inequalities in Health before Black.' *Contemporary British History* 16 (3): 81–104.

Whipple, Amy C. 2010. '"Into Every Home, into Every Body": Organicism and Anti-statism in the British Anti-fluoridation Movement, 1952–1960.' *Twentieth Century British History* 21 (3): 330–49.

Williams, Raymond. 1973. *Keywords: A Vocabulary of Culture and Society*. London: 4th Estate.

Yarwood, J., K. Noakes, D. Kennedy, H. Campbell, and D. Salisbury. 2005. 'Tracking Mothers Attitudes to Childhood Immunisation 1991–2001.' *Vaccine* 23 (48–49): 5670–87.

Young, Michael, and Peter Wilmott. 2013. *Family and Kinship in East London*. Oxon: Routledge.

CHAPTER 4

Speaking Back

Abstract In this chapter, we consider how the public or certain publics were able to 'speak back' to public health, to challenge its practices and ideologies. We focus on three types of speaking back. The first involved resistance. This could be active, as in the rejection of public health initiatives, or more passive, such as hesitancy or reluctance to engage. The second form of speaking back consisted of complaints made to public health authorities. These included complaints about being surveyed and complaints made to local public health officials. The third form of speaking back involved reinterpretation or appropriation of public health recommendations and communications by sections of the public. We argue that the public, or at least parts of it, in specific contexts, had agency.

Keywords Resistance · Complaint · Surveys · Health education · Vaccination · Lay epidemiology · Coronary heart disease

The public in post-war Britain was not an inert object. Members of the public, as individuals and as groups, could 'speak back' to public health authorities. In this chapter we examine the various forms that speaking back could take, and the scenarios in which this took place. We focus on three principal types of speaking back. The first involved resistance, whereby members of the public deliberately opposed or reacted against public health

A. Mold et al., *Placing the Public in Public Health in Post-War Britain, 1948–2012*, Medicine and Biomedical Sciences in Modern History,
https://doi.org/10.1007/978-3-030-18685-2_4

policies and practices. Such resistance could be active, as, for example, in anti-vaccination campaigns. Other kinds of public resistance could be more passive, encompassing reluctance or hesitancy to engage with public health initiatives. The second form of speaking back can be found in complaints made by the public to public health authorities. These included complaints about being surveyed and complaints made to local public health officials. The third type of speaking back involved reinterpretation or appropriation of public health recommendations and communications by sections of the public. Some members of the public were able to turn public health messages on their head, and present different interpretations or readings of these. By focusing on three areas we are excluding some other forms of speaking back. These include instances where the public made specific demands for public health initiatives like vaccination or screening (Millward 2017a; Lowy 2011). Such demands aligned with the goals of public health policy and practitioners, even if they were not realised at the time. In this chapter, we are interested in how the public offered a challenge to the practice of public health and its outlook.

All of these different types of speaking back indicate that the public, or at least certain parts of it, and in specific contexts, had agency. In this chapter we examine the settings and scenarios where the public was able to speak back. This encompasses public responses to public health practices like vaccination and the survey, as well as the different ways in which the public engaged with health education. We also pay attention to who was doing the speaking back. Often, the publics most able to speak back to public health were those in the most privileged social position. Middle-class white men, for example, were more likely to complain about being included in public health surveys than other social groups. Yet, speaking back can be found among more marginalised groups too. Women, and particularly mothers, were heavily involved in resistance towards vaccination. Working-class responses to health education messages about Coronary Heart Disease (CHD) displayed a reluctance to take these entirely at face value. Young people were able to actively reinterpret anti-drug campaign materials. Public health practitioners and policymakers, then, encountered a public that was far from inert.

1 Resistance

Public resistance, or the refusal to accept or comply with public health practices and policies could be characterised as either 'active' or 'passive'. Active resistance involved the visible rejection of initiatives such as vaccination or refusing to participate in public health surveys. Yet, the public also engaged in more passive ways of resisting public health authorities. This included being slow to take up programmes like vaccination or being reluctant to talk to surveyors. The distinction between 'active' and 'passive' resistance was often blurred, but such a categorisation draws attention to some of the recognisable and less obvious ways the public opposed different public health initiatives.

1.1 Active Resistance

Active resistance towards immunisation was nothing new in the field of public health. Objections to these procedures in Britain go back to the introduction of inoculation in the eighteenth century (Eriksen 2016). Once variolation and, later, vaccination were brought into local and national public health programmes during the nineteenth century, older concerns about scientific, economic, cultural or religious validity persisted. Objections became openly framed around the political consideration of the rights of the individual versus the need to protect the collective (Colgrove 2006). This became increasingly fraught after the introduction of compulsory vaccination in 1840. The Anti-vaccination League and protests associated with the movement led to the end of compulsory vaccination by the close of the nineteenth century (Durbach 2005).

This legacy made successive twentieth-century British governments hesitant to impose immunisation upon the population. For example, during the Second World War the diphtheria immunisation programme was based on advertising, education and persuasion. It was successful in combatting the disease, despite lobbying from anti-vaccination and anti-vivisection groups. These organisations claimed that diphtheria immunisation did not work, was unsafe, should not be imposed on parents, was a waste of taxpayer's money, and relied upon manufacturing techniques that were cruel to horses (Correspondence and ephemera). Parents nonetheless presented their children for the procedure in large numbers. Partly this was because they feared the effects of the disease, a well-known hazard in the 1940s. Also, as the programme progressed, it became clear both through official statistics and lived experience that diphtheria was becoming less common, immunised children were less likely to get the disease, and, if they did, they were much more likely to survive it. The response from parents, coupled with the legacy of nineteenth-century anti-vaccination sentiment, meant that in 1948 the Vaccination Acts were repealed and future immunisation schemes were based on central government funding, education and persuasion rather than compulsion. By the time pertussis (whooping cough) and poliomyelitis vaccinations were added to the national vaccination schedule in the 1950s, anti-vaccination organisations had little reach.

While blanket anti-vaccinationism may not have concerned the Ministry of Health and its successors in the post-war period, campaigns against specific vaccines during moments of crisis did emerge. In the 1970s, reports that the pertussis vaccine might cause brain damage led to a significant decrease in uptake (Baker 2003). As parents made a conscious choice to avoid the vaccine, the campaign led by the Association of Parents of Vaccine Damaged Children successfully lobbied for social security payments to children where it could be shown that a vaccine probably led to serious disability. While the initial catalyst for the campaign had been reports of brain damage, it gained traction in the specific political climate of the 1970s. Parental trust in the medical profession had been dented by the thalidomide scandal. Moreover, debates over social security and collectivised risk for vaccine damage were magnified by the ongoing financial crisis and examinations of the viability of a comprehensive welfare state (Millward 2017b). The measles-mumps-rubella vaccine (MMR) crisis at the turn of the millennium was similarly a product of its time. Reports that MMR might cause autism—and that the government or medical profession might have made fatal mistakes—were believable following the scandals around bovine spongiform encephalopathy (BSE, or 'mad cow disease'), contaminated blood, Alder Hey hospital and Bristol heart operations (Hargreaves et al. 2003). With both pertussis and MMR, new approaches to communicating with the public helped the government promote the mounting evidence that the vaccines were safe and that the science underpinning the vaccine-sceptic claims was flawed. But uptake took many years to recover, leading to outbreaks of the diseases that were significantly larger than if vaccination rates had remained at pre-crisis levels (Dobson 2008; Baker 2003).

A new feature of anti-vaccinationism from the 1990s onwards was the ability to form and mobilise internet communities, which were able to disseminate their literature to a much wider audience than was previously possible. This created a new challenge for public health authorities. The long-standing regime of education and persuasion did not produce linear progress in achieving universal acceptance of vaccination, as the pertussis and MMR crises showed. Still, active opposition to (or, at least, refusal of) vaccines remained relatively uncommon. Over 91% of children under the age of two received the MMR vaccine in 2016–2017 (NHS 2017). Improvements in surveillance and follow up made a significant impact on increasing vaccination uptake since the 1980s, but practical developments alone cannot explain widespread public acceptance of vaccination. According to Jacob Heller, most of the population believes a particular narrative about vaccination: vaccines work, they are safe and advanced nations provide them as a sign of their modernity (Heller 2008). Individual vaccines at specific times, however, can produce opposition to which governments are forced to react. Vaccination, then, was both a site of active resistance and acceptance on the part of the public.

Active resistance to public health policies and practices was not confined to anti-vaccinationism. One of the most effective ways to 'speak back' to public health was to not speak at all. The refusal to participate in public health surveys registered the non-respondent's dissatisfaction with the process, but also held the potential to jeopardise the study by making it unrepresentative; threatening the generalisability and validity of the results (Robinson et al. 2007). For this reason, studies run since the emergence of representative sampling worked hard to minimise refusals: developing persuasive information sheets; crafting carefully inoffensive questions; sometimes providing incentives; and concentrating on improving interviewer rapport; among other strategies (Dohrenwend and Dohrenwend 1969; Mitchell et al. 2007). The silent nature of this form of resistance also makes it difficult to trace and understand. The Government Social Survey (GSS) department was proud to note in 1949 that 'only about two people in every 100 refuse to cooperate … and 95 per cent of the people spoken to express their willingness to cooperate in future enquiries', but held little information on that two per cent, who they were and what motivated their resistance to the survey (Complaints Received from Members of the Public Interviewed by S.S. Investigators, 1949).

In his study of mental health in Harlow across 1959 and 1960, researcher Sidney Chave made an effort to collect information on why people refused to participate. In his diaries we can see some of the reasons given by non-respondents to the survey interviewers and recorded by Chave third-hand. Early in the survey, one interviewer was refused twice on the same day by 'a man who said he and his family were all healthy and did not care about anyone else' and a 'GPO [General Post Office] shift worker who said he was not interested' (Sidney Chave, Research Diary—The Health Survey, 6 May 1959). These refusals seemed to indicate a misunderstanding of the purpose of the survey, or apathy, rather than overt disapproval. They were read this way by Chave, who 'drafted a persuasive letter' to be given to 'potential refusers' the next day (Sidney Chave, Research Diary—The Health Survey, 7 May 1959). Despite this, small numbers of people continued to refuse. In the same month, Chave recorded the following account of three refusals in one household:

> Large household: … 8 children. Very dirty. Wife interviewed … Husband big lout, foul-mouthed, kept interrupting, full of complaints about [Harlow] … Got nothing else to do but go to bed/have children. Would not be interviewed, then made an appointment for Sunday – but when interviewer arrived kept her talking – full of complaints but would not be interviewed. Refused to let her see his teenage children. (Sidney Chave, Research Diary—The Health Survey, 22 May 1959)

This account of resistance to the process of being surveyed says less about why this man refused on behalf of himself and his children, and more about how Chave and his interviewing team viewed non-respondents. While the previous refusals were framed in terms of 'apathy', this refusal to participate was seen as part of a series of inappropriate behaviours; from keeping a dirty house and having too many children, to wasting the interviewer's time by inviting her back only to refuse her on a second occasion. Despite the work put in to persuading people to cooperate, participation was treated as the norm, and an aspect of good citizenship. The expansion of the welfare state in the immediate post-war period brought with it a number of rights to access public services, including healthcare, but these were balanced with social responsibilities (Marshall 1992). Taking part in a survey could be construed as one of the duties of social citizenship. Indeed, refusal to participate was seen as not just a problem for the study, but a potential signifier of wider issues. Regarding this particular set of refusals, Chave noted that his interviewer had been 'told by neighbours this family [was] a cause of much local disturbance' (Sidney Chave, Research Diary—The Health Survey, 22 May 1959).

Such interpretations of refusal, and the people who refused, reflected the nature of social research at the time. Sociologist Mike Savage argues that in Britain a 'gentlemanly social science' concerned with 'mapping populations and separating out groups according to their moral worth and respectability' prevailed well into the 1950s (Savage 2010, 19, 12). Savage finds evidence of this 'moralising and medicalising tradition' in the field notes for Elizabeth Bott's influential 1957 study *Family and Social Network*, in which the respondents' 'psychological emotions and social states were extensively discussed' by the research team (Savage 2010, 96). We can see both tendencies, 'moralising' and 'medicalising', in Chave's Harlow study. By the end of the study Chave, influenced by Ann Cartwright's 1959 article on 'non-cooperators' in Oxhey, began to see non-compliance with his survey as a potential symptom of the mental health issues he was investigating (Cartwright 1959; Sidney Chave, Research Diary—Collecting the GP Records, 4 January 1960). Chave delved into the medical records of those who refused, and found in their histories a slightly greater 'prevalence of nervous symptoms' than in the average population (Taylor and Chave 1964, 197–98). In the 1950s, those who refused to participate had the potential to be seen as deviant or unwell.

However, across the post-war period, refusals could also be viewed as an alternative form of engagement. Rather than pointing towards a recalcitrant, apathetic or deviant public they contribute to our understanding of where people's boundaries lay in relation to participation. The National Survey of Health and Development, a birth cohort study which began in 1946, and is still surveying its members today, has monitored its loss to follow-up over the decades. In 1992, the then study director, Michael Wadsworth, noted that 'between ages 15 and 36 years permanent refusals of contact rose, most steeply than between 31 and 36 years'. Wadsworth suggested that the rise in refusals at 36 years could be attributable to the 'introduction of measurements of blood pressure and respiratory function, and the first adult measures of height and weight' in the study. For some study members, this was asking too much. On the other hand, the 'greatest source of loss at 43–44 years was temporary refusal … when personal or family problems made it impossible for the study member to be interviewed or measured on this occasion', suggesting that some refusals were merely a deferral of participation (Wadsworth et al. 1992, 301, 303). Similarly, the most recent round of the National Survey of Sexual Attitudes and Lifestyles (Natsal) allowed participants to 'choose not to answer' any questions they were uncomfortable with. Surprisingly, the surveyors found that less than three per cent refused to answer 'the most sensitive questions' about sex but that twenty per cent refused to reveal their income (Soazig 2014). What people have refused to answer and when has been more frequently recorded by surveyors than why. Perhaps more telling is the way that researchers have responded to refusals. As studies moved away from the 'gentlemanly social science' model and began to view participants as individuals with rights and boundaries, it became possible to view refusal not just as active resistance, but as an alternative form of engagement to be managed accordingly (Marsh 1985, 215).

1.2 *Passive Resistance*

More passive forms of resistance, such as being reluctant, apathetic or slow to engage with public health policies and practices, were also exhibited by the public at various times and in a range of different ways. Vaccination, for example, was not just met with active defiance, but more passive resistance too. As discussed earlier, the British government moved away from compulsory vaccination over the course of the twentieth century. The prioritisation of education and persuasion necessarily put the emphasis on individual choice to either vaccinate or not. In the post-war period, significant energy was spent on investigating why certain parents 'chose' not to vaccinate their children and what could be done about it. A common explanation was 'apathy'. A sharp decline in uptake of diphtheria immunisation in 1950 was blamed on apathetic mothers. Public health authorities believed that a generation that had benefited from the successes of the anti-diphtheria programme now no-longer feared the disease and so were not making 'sufficient' effort to present their children for the procedure (A message from the Chief Medical Officer, December 1950). The lack of direct opposition to immunisation, as shown, for example, in the high number of permission slips returned for vaccinations in schools, indicated that parents were not against vaccination per se (Diphtheria Prophylaxis: Publicity Campaign for Immunisation). Yet, they did not present in sufficient enough numbers to satisfy the Ministry of Health, hampering efforts to continue to see year-on-year decreases in morbidity and mortality.

This hinterland between out-right opposition and compliance was shown in other vaccination schemes. Uptake of smallpox vaccination had been in decline since the effective end of compulsion in the 1890s (Rafferty et al. 2018). Advertising efforts led to some recovery in the 1950s, but routine infant vaccination rates remained stubbornly low. However, when local areas were at direct risk of an epidemic of smallpox, long queues snaked around the streets near the Medical Officer of Health's (MOH) clinic demanding emergency vaccination (Douglas and Edgar 1962). Similarly, the Minister of Health was disgruntled when the death of footballer Jeff Hall from polio in 1959 saw a sharp increase in young adults presenting for polio vaccination, creating localised shortages. The Minister argued that if the population had complied with requests to register beforehand rather than being 'apathetic' about the threat from these diseases, the surges in demand would not have put so much pressure on supplies (HC Deb, 27 April 1959).

Although surges in demand were seen as problematic, the Ministry spent little time analysing why parents made (in its eyes) the 'right' decision with vaccination. However, it showed awareness of structural factors that may have prevented parents from being compliant. Officials understood, for instance, that parents were more likely to present their children for vaccination when it was convenient. Diphtheria immunisation rates were much higher among school pupils—where vaccination required no further action on the part of the parent other than returning a permission slip—than among pre-schoolers where parents would have to present their children to a local clinic. Middle-class parents were also more likely to vaccinate, partly due to education but also because they had more capacity to take the time and effort to present their children. Over successive years, the Ministry introduced a number of initiatives to make vaccination easier for parents to access. This included the development of combined vaccines to reduce the number of clinic trips, moving vaccination away from the MOH's clinic to the GP's surgery, providing sophisticated automated reminder systems, compiling detailed statistics about uptake, undertaking regular surveys to monitor parental attitudes, and improving educational technologies to convince parents that the inconvenience of vaccination was far outweighed by its benefits to the individual and society (Silcock and Ratcliffe 1996; Begg et al. 1989; Yarwood et al. 2005).

Recent crises across the world have led to reappraisals of how vaccination programmes work and why publics make certain choices. To some, these crises are 'inevitable'. As vaccines become 'victims of their own success', parents see stories of adverse events and come to question their utility. Subsequent outbreaks of the disease (combined with education efforts) reassert the vaccine's reputation, leading eventually to the disease's eradication (Chen and Hibbs 1998). Others have focused on decision making, both in the 'positive' and 'negative' sense. Work on 'vaccine confidence' looks at a range of factors for why parents make vaccination decisions. It posits that few people are adamant that they will always or never vaccinate, and that most are somewhere in between on a vaccine-by-vaccine basis (Larson et al. 2015). These explanations acknowledge the heterogeneity of public opinion and belief. They derive explicitly from the supposed 'lessons from history' of crises such as pertussis and MMR in the UK in the 1970s and 2000s (Berridge et al. 2011). But such explanations are also historically contingent responses to the politics of global public health in the twenty-first century. World Health Organization vaccination targets, for example, demand that 95% of children receive MMR before the age of 5. Thus, states and public health organisations are under pressure to secure near-universal compliance with vaccination policy. New metrics for confidence and compliance are therefore a key technology for identifying and combatting vaccine 'hesitancy' (Larson et al. 2014). This removes some of the accusatory undertones of the 'apathy' framing from earlier periods, emphasising choice rather than a lack of adequate care. At the same time, public health officials' focus on reducing risk and ensuring compliance with medical guidelines mean that people that make the 'wrong' choices are still seen as deviant.

A slightly different form of passive resistance to public health can be identified in relation to the public health survey. Members of the public sometimes participated in public health surveys reluctantly. Tracing reluctance in the historical record is particularly difficult as it was rarely identified by surveyors at the time. For example, in May 1951, a woman from Croydon wrote to the GSS to express her dissatisfaction with being surveyed by the Wartime Survey of Sickness. She wrote that although she was 'very busy and pressed for time', she had participated in the survey because the interviewer had been 'very insistent'. However, she had resisted the survey in the only way left available to her, by lying: 'I am now glad to say that all [answers] were not true (I felt irritated and puzzled at the call)'. From this account, one might expect the interviewer to have realised that something was wrong. Yet when questioned, the interviewer was apologetic but replied that she did 'not recall having had any difficulty at this address' (Complaints Received from Members of the Public Interviewed by S.S. Investigators, 8 May 1951). This was not an isolated incident. In July 1951, an ex-army officer wrote to the GSS to say that he too had felt pressured into answering despite his reluctance: the interviewer's 'methods bore a slight resemblance to high-pressure salesmanship, a detective showing his search warrant, and a bailiff trying to gain admittance to a house'. Once again, the interviewer in question was unaware that there had been a problem: 'These people seemed to be so friendly at the time of the interview'. The interviewer also expressed confusion as to why 'people who do not wish to be interviewed … do not "refuse" when … the opportunity has been given freely and pleasantly to do so' (Complaints Received from Members of the Public Interviewed by S.S. Investigators, 14 July 1951).

Some did refuse, but others evidently felt unable to and sought to resist the survey in more subtle ways.

As Natsal's qualitative research into their survey methods has shown, lying to surveyors is an unusual form of resistance. Once people agree to take part in the research, as Clifton Soazig notes, there often 'seems no point in giving inaccurate answers' (Soazig 2014). Rather than lying outright however, giving evasive answers was another form of subtle resistance available to survey participants. The final question of a 1944 GSS inquiry into venereal disease (VD) asked participants, 'what else do you think should be done to stamp out VD apart from publicity?' Only fifty-six per cent of respondents made suggestions, with thirty-nine per cent recording a 'don't know/no ideas' response and five per cent making 'no answer' at all. GSS researchers found that 'analyses by education, income, sex, marital status and age' showed 'that certain groups of people have more constructive suggestions to make than others'. Sixty-seven per cent of men made suggestions compared with forty-eight per cent of women, and seventy-three per cent on a 'higher income' did compared with fifty-four per cent on a 'lower income' (Wilson and Barker 1944, 53–54). For the most part, this may have been reflective of knowledge and education levels, and of confidence in one's views. But it is worth noting that this inquiry was carried out in factories and asked workers to 'sacrifice' their time even when they were 'working on piece-rates' (Box and Thomas 1944). Rather than being ignorant or apathetic, some people, male or female, might have answered 'don't know' to get back to work more quickly. It is possible they were conscious of their lost wages, embarrassed to be asked about VD at work, or unwilling to reveal the extent of their knowledge of sensitive subjects to an interviewer (Fisher 2008, 6, 67). In this light, claims of ignorance could have been utilised as a less confrontational form of resistance more accessible and familiar to some than outright refusal or complaint, and could be read as evidence of survey reluctance. Resistance to public health policies and practices like surveys, could, therefore, take a number of forms and move along a continuum from 'active' to 'passive'.

2 Complaints

One of the most obvious, although problematic, ways the public could speak back to public health was by complaining. Although rare, complaints offer useful insights into public perceptions and attitudes that can be otherwise difficult to grasp. The philosopher Julian Baggini argues that complaining is more than moaning, that 'there is value in reflecting on what our complaints say about ourselves' (Baggini 2008, 3, 128). Reflections are possible because complaints require 'going public'. John Clarke suggests that whereas a grievance can remain private, the process of submitting a complaint to the relevant authority and investigation procedure makes it inherently public and leaves a record. Complaints represent a 'hinterland' of 'anxieties, doubts and frustrations'; the public articulation of private grumblings shared by many people (Clarke 2014, 261). They tell us not only what some objected to, but what other members of the public acquiesced to and the conditions they tolerated. There is also value in noting which people were able to make complaints. While the very act of complaining results in the creation of a public record and can be read as an expression of a public feeling, albeit a formally constructed and unusually vocal one, complaints are often individual and can reveal how different members of the public and sections of society were able to engage with public health (Clarke 2014, 262). Examination of complaints made to public health authorities reveals shared points of tension in the relationships between members of the public and public health and can shed light on other more subtle forms of 'speaking back' such as reluctance, apathy and hesitance.

2.1 *Complaints and the Survey*

For Tom Crook, modern public health involved multiple agents: experts and administrators matched an active and accountable public, all of whom were both 'objects and subjects of power' (Crook 2016, 16–17). The survey offers an excellent arena within which to observe how certain sections of the public were more able than others to 'speak back' to public health. This points to hierarchies of expertise and the relationships between different publics and public health. In sampling the whole adult population of England and Wales, the GSS's 1943–1952 Survey of Sickness engaged a broad public in public health research. Some of those surveyed had not previously experienced the scrutiny of the state in their homes and had perhaps not recognised themselves as being a 'public' of public health before. The Ministry of Health still deemed it largely 'inappropriate' to focus on men up until the end of the 1950s (Berridge 2007, 188). Men who had experienced medical surveillance in the army could baulk at attempts to survey them at home and in peace time (Newlands 2014, 27). Sections of the public were able to wield more power than others, but what the Survey of Sickness complaints show us is that the role of the public in public health was not just varied, but up for negotiation. Men and the middle classes, newly aware of their role as the subjects of public health research, were able and willing to construct complaints, and in doing so affected change on the survey process. As Clarke argues, when institutional practices are transgressive of public–private boundaries, institutions expend a lot of effort to mitigate the transgression by 'establishing the notion of consent—and the maintenance of legitimacy in the face of dissent' (Clarke 2014, 263). This was evident in the response of the GSS to some criticisms.

As mentioned in Chapter 3, a frequent topic of complaint was from men concerned with being asked to give information about their salary. One man expressed shock at being asked questions of a 'very personal nature ... my age ... my employment ... my SALARY' (Complaints Received from Members of the Public Interviewed by S.S. Investigators, 3 May 1951). Another could not understand why such information was needed: 'please let me know what connection ... there is between my daughter's health and my occupation and Income?' (Complaints Received from Members of the Public Interviewed by S.S. Investigators, 9 May 1951). But even those who understood the necessity of putting health in a social context, or trusted that there was a reason, expressed annoyance with having to reveal their income in person and on the doorstep. To combat this the GSS issued each interviewer with a card printed with income categories so that the survey subject could 'indicate... his income' non-verbally (Survey of Sickness: Instructions to Interviewers). The GSS met what Clarke terms the 'modest demands of respect, dignity and recognition' articulated by its new, male, vocal public. These demands were 'highly individual and personal', yet, when shared, evoked 'norms of social and organisational conduct' and questioned the practices of the survey (Clarke 2014, 268).

The complaints received—largely around issues of privacy, liberty, waste of time or government money, and the conduct of interviewers—were often reflected in wider public discourse, especially in the popular press (*Daily Mail*, 2 August 1940, 8 November 1941; *Daily Express*, 27 July 1944, 3; 17 November 1949; *Sunday Express*, 11 June 1950; *The Times*, 30 June 1944, 5 February 1946, 10 December 1948). For example, some people writing to the GSS used the popular press shorthand 'snooper' to complain about interviewers (Complaints Received from Members of the Public Interviewed by S.S. Investigators, Fieldworker Report, 19 July 1950; Beers 2006). Other sections of the public who were not represented in the complaints may have held similar grievances. In the case of the Survey of Sickness, very few complaints were from working-class women. As explained above, these women may have resisted the survey in their own ways; through using 'don't know' as a quick answer, or deliberately misleading survey staff, but the survey's perception of them as ignorant of matters outside the home and their families often obscured such forms of resistance. As a result, they had little influence on the survey process ("Anatomy of the 'Don't Knows'," December 1947).

The complaints made against the Survey of Sickness reveal a complex set of relationships between different sections of the public and the British state; ones of power and prejudice. As Sara Ahmed notes, a complaint that identifies and challenges 'abuses of power teaches us about power' (Ahmed, n.d.). Complaints about privacy and liberty suggested that for some people there was a definite limit to what information the state should ask from citizens and how it should collect that information. On a case by case basis people struck a careful balance 'between rights and benefits', relinquishing privacy only when they considered the exchange fair (Vincent 2016, 101). Complaints about wasted resources indicated that members of the public felt they had a stake in how public money was spent, and that the survey was not a good use of it. These complaints could overlap, as one woman articulated: 'it is an absolute intrusion and an indignity—as well as a waste of Government money' (Health Index Survey: General Correspondence, 29 July 1948). People also valued their own time and contested public health authorities' claims to it, as one man wrote: 'my house was invaded without notice and I only realised when it was finished that I had been participating in yet another waste of public money and private time' (Complaints Received from Members of the Public Interviewed by S.S. Investigators, 21 July 1950). Last, complaints about interviewers suggested that the authority of the state was contingent on people recognising it and that this was influenced by existing prejudices and power structures.

While some of these complaints were context specific, such as those drawing on people's experiences in the Second World War—'I cling rather obstinately to the idea … of freedom for which I fought during the recent war'—others have occurred in surveys since (Complaints Received from Members of the Public Interviewed by S.S. Investigators, 9 December 1947). Yet, just as GSS director Louis Moss wrote in 1951: 'I do not accept complaints as inevitable for <u>any</u> kind of work. Our experience over the years has shown that we can, by appropriate care, reduce complaints to insignificant proportions', researchers working on public health surveys increasingly accepted the need to make the process as tolerable as possible for participants (Complaints Received from Members of the Public Interviewed by S.S. Investigators, 29 November 1951). As public health evolved in the post-war period, influenced by the ideology of social medicine, everyone became a participant in public health. But just as the role of public health was up for negotiation, so too was the role of the public, especially for those with the leverage to negotiate.

2.2 *Complaints to Medical Officers of Health*

The survey was not the only avenue open to those wishing to complain about aspects of public health policy and practice. Local public health officials encountered the public at various junctures and such interactions offered opportunities for complaint, both formal and informal. The MOH was the official in charge of public health at the local level from the nineteenth century until the scrapping of the post following the reorganisation of health services in 1973. The ability to complain about 'nuisances' to the MOH was not unique to the post-war period, but after the establishment of the NHS in 1948, the MOH retained responsibility for various aspects of environmental health about which the public could complain (Crook 2016). Indeed, the lack of formal complaints procedures within the NHS until the 1980s meant that those wishing to complain about certain aspects of public health were perhaps better served than those wanting to complain about treatment in hospital or general practice (Mold 2015, 69–93). Residents dissatisfied with the condition of food purchased from local shops and other outlets could complain to the MOH, who would then investigate. Such complaints, their pursuit and eventual outcome, featured heavily in the annual reports produced by the MOH. In his report of 1955, for instance, the MOH for Surbiton recorded complaints from members of the public about mould found in sausages, meat pies and Eccles cakes, as well as a wasp in a rusk (MOH for Surbiton, Annual Report 1955, 43–44). If such complaints were found to be valid, MOH could take various courses of action, including writing warning letters to food producers, or even bringing legal proceedings, potentially resulting in a fine or possible closure of the premises. The public could also complain to the MOH about other nuisances, such as noise. In 1962, the MOH for Woolwich noted that 'Noise continues to give some residents cause for complaint, and the Public Health Inspectors made 50 inspections connected with noise complaints during the year under review'. Of particular concern were chimes from ice-cream vendors' vans during the summer months (MOH for Woolwich, Annual Report 1962, 22). Various other noise complaints ranging from crowing cockerels, to noisy 'jive clubs', hammering at all night garages, and factories blowing off steam late at night were dealt with by informal action. Banal as these complaints may seem, they indicated a willingness on the part of both the public and public health officials to take seriously the concerns of the local population and a desire to improve conditions for all.

Other, more informal, opportunities for complaint also arose, and could hint at wider concerns held by members of the public. One such scenario was during the public exhibitions run by MOH. These exhibitions were intended to educate the public about various aspects of public health, including topics such as food hygiene, smokeless fuels and the dangers of tobacco (Mold 2018). The exhibitions offered a rare chance for direct interaction between members of the public and the staff of the public health department. At an exhibition arranged by the MOH for Stepney in 1950 visitors were able to ask questions and complain to officials staffing the show. The MOH asserted that such complaints were frequently 'irrelevant and turned on housing and personal economic difficulties' (MOH for Stepney, Annual Report 1950, 64). While other MOH went out of their way to solicit the views of the public, they too did not always get the responses they desired. In 1959, the MOH for Camberwell conducted a survey to find out what the public thought of the borough's 'health propaganda'. Although some pertinent concerns were raised, the MOH grumbled that comments made by the public 'often reflected the particular grievances of the respondents, such as complaints about litter on waste land, and inadequate housing' (MOH for Camberwell, Annual Report 1959, 13–14). The public could use such fora as places to raise issues that concerned them, even if MOH thought these to be irrelevant or outside their brief. Indeed, the active use of such means by the public to complain raises the possibility that the public were able to use public health mechanisms to do more than simply respond, but rather to actively reinvent these for their own ends.

3 Reinterpretation and Appropriation

Some public health measures were open to reinterpretation or even appropriation by the public. This involved more than passive or active rejection or acceptance, but a concerted effort to change the meaning or purpose of such policies and practices. This could include reading public health campaign material in the opposite way to that which was intended, or even inverting the meaning of this and deliberately reworking such material to produce a different message. In this way, the public (or certain parts of it) was able to create its own meanings and ascribe these to public health concepts and initiatives.

3.1 Letters to Whitehall

Public health surveys were designed to think of and deal with the public as a collective, but participants could turn this on its head, and use the survey to explore aspects of their own health. The Whitehall study was a longitudinal health survey of male civil servants carried out between 1967 and 1970. The study screened over 18,000 men aged between 45 and 60 years primarily for cardiovascular and respiratory conditions, with follow up dietary and exercise studies performed on samples of the cohort. The follow-up studies necessitated further communication between study participants and researcher Geoffrey Rose, whether he was sending them dietary questionnaires to complete or instructing them on how to use the pedometer sent to them in the post. Although the majority of participants completed their postal questionnaires without incident, a number used the opportunity to ask questions and engage with the study in ways which reinterpreted its purpose or appropriated it for their own ends.

Although the instructions accompanying the dietary survey questionnaire made it clear to the participants that they need only include a note if 'the amount or type of food you ate on any of these days was unusual for you', many wrote back to explain how they were in some way 'unusual' themselves, warning Rose that they may not be representative (Correspondence regarding dietary habits postal survey). As one man wrote, 'we have most irregular eating habits and what is "fairly typical" to me is probably otherwise to others … I feel that I do not well fit into an average category but if there are not too many of a similar nature in your sample it should not unbalance it' (Correspondence regarding dietary habits postal survey, 3 June 1969). While some men seemed worried that they might prejudice the survey results, skewing Rose's understanding of 'the diet of the group as a whole', others took the opportunity to either assert a sense of individual subjectivity or ask for reassurance or advice. Foucault argued that in research the interview acts as a 'device for producing confessional accounts', allowing 'subjects to self-produce their subjectivity' (Savage 2010, 165). With this in mind, it could be argued that for some participants in the Whitehall study, the questionnaire proved too narrow a form for self-expression. These men wrote to Rose to share more details about their lives. One man advised Rose that his questionnaire was 'certainly not designed to help vegetarians', before launching into a description of a diet largely consisting of dried fruit, salad, vegetables and eggs (Correspondence regarding dietary habits postal survey). Another tried to explain his somewhat erratic eating habits: 'since I have been widowed I eat when I want to and at no special time. I trust this will help' (Correspondence regarding dietary habits postal survey, 15 July 1970). In both these accounts we can see what Sarah Igo calls the 'subtle conversion of individual experiences into social scientific data' (Igo 2009, 282). These men were keen to share their stories and did so with an understanding that this added information was 'useful to science', whether or not Rose ultimately took note of it (Savage 2010, 165).

For others, engagement in scientific research could be an opportunity to seek 'expert assurances' about their relative 'normality' (Igo 2009, 279). As one man wrote, 'my friends and colleagues seem to find my eating habits erratic and amusing. If they are medically unusual I would welcome your views' (Correspondence regarding dietary habits postal survey, 21 January 1969). Others' anxieties were prompted by the study itself: 'Naturally I am … slightly perturbed at the inference that my survey medical check revealed some peculiarity that evoked further interest' (Correspondence regarding dietary habits postal survey). Another respondent was at pains to check that he was receiving the necessary medical advice: 'I assume that I do not come within the category "certain medical conditions" which might be associated with "special eating habits" … If the contrary is the case I hope that either my medical practitioner or myself will be advised accordingly' (Correspondence regarding dietary habits postal survey). Rose replied to this man and the others who sent similar enquiries, explaining that they had not been selected for any specific reason, but that their contributions would put the study in a 'better position to help those individuals who are not fit' (Correspondence regarding dietary habits postal survey). As well as pleas for reassurance, in these interactions we can see the transactional element to participation in the study. These men understood that through their full participation they would gain early notice of any health problems they might have and were keen to make sure this was met. Others took it further, asking directly for advice: 'If any recommendations issue as a result of your survey I should be most grateful if I might be told what they are. I try reasonably hard to reduce my weight but achieve poor results, yet I feel that I do not over eat' (Correspondence regarding dietary habits postal survey, 26 January 1969). While indicative of an understanding of participation as a two-way exchange, this letter anticipating the results of the study reminds us that the individuals who took part were also members of the public who could stand to benefit from the knowledge produced. As Igo wrote in her work on American public opinion surveys, 'surveys are a peculiar sort of social investigation in which the public is simultaneously object, participant, and audience' (Igo 2009, 4). The men who took part in the Whitehall study and its subsidiary surveys participated as asked, but they were not passive subjects. They each brought their own motivations and agendas to the study, and through speaking back in various ways embodied one of the tensions inherent to public health research, that of 'being an individual and being a statistic'(Igo 2009, 282).

3.2 *Health Education*

The relationship of the individual to the tools of public health authorities and their capacity to turn these to their own advantage is powerfully illustrated by health education. Mass media public health campaigns were first contemplated in the mid-1960s, but only really began to take shape in the 1970s. Such campaigns were open to active reinterpretation or appropriation by those that saw them. An excellent example is offered by the 1985–1986 'Heroin Screws You Up' campaign. Prior to 1980s, there was very little health education messaging specifically on drugs. In large part, this was because health educators and drug experts believed that drug education would be counter-productive, indeed it might actually encourage young people to use drugs (Manning 2013). However, a significant rise in the number of heroin users during the early 1980s, and an ensuing moral panic about drug use, prompted the government to launch an anti-heroin campaign. The campaign, designed by the advertising agency Yellowhammer for the Central Office of Information (COI), consisted of a series of images reproduced on posters, in newspapers and in magazines as well as two brief TV commercials. All of the images featured young people, supposedly heroin users, in various states of distress. All were pale, with dark circles under their eyes, often with dirty-looking hair, and of a generally dishevelled appearance. The text surrounding the images listed some of the likely consequences of heroin use including addiction, sickness and loss of control. An evaluation of the campaign carried out for the COI found that it had a high degree of penetration: nearly all of the respondents recalled having seen either the TV advertisements, the posters or press images. Moreover, the research suggested that there had been significant change before and after the campaign in relation to awareness about the health risks associated with heroin use. Respondents also reported being less likely to take heroin if offered it by a friend after the campaign (Research Bureau International 1986).

Yet, the Heroin Screws You Up campaign came in for widespread criticism from those working in the drugs field, the wider media and even an internal Department of Health and Social Security review. Some critics saw the tone of the campaign as making use of fear tactics to scare young people into not using drugs, something which could increase the stigmatisation around drugs and drug users. There were also concerns that such images would not be credible to those young people more familiar with drugs (Rhodes 1990). Worse still, from a prevention standpoint, scare tactics might actually have encouraged young people to use drugs as an act of rebellion (Falk-Whynes 1991). Other critics pointed out that the campaign was too broadly targeted, unlikely to achieve behaviour or attitude change and that attitudes towards drugs were influenced by a range of other media, and embedded within broader cultural and social structures and values (Hansen 1985; Woodcock 1986; Power 1989). Indeed, the public response to the campaign seemed to indicate that it did more than miss the mark. Some youths deliberately appropriated the campaign and its imagery. There were numerous reports that young people took the poster or the magazine and newspaper advertisements and put them up on their bedroom walls. In 1989, Barry Sheerman (Labour MP for Huddersfield East) told the House of Commons that 'The rather effete young man in the heroin posters became a pin-up for some young girls'. Health Minister David Mellor responded that this was an allegation that had never been proven (HC Deb, 8 December 1989) (Fig. 4.1).

It is hard to say for certain whether the Heroin Screws You Up posters really became teenage pin-ups, but the imagery the campaign used was open to wider cultural appropriation or even reappropriation. This is an example of what media studies theorists describe as the 'polysemic' nature of 'texts': that these are open to multiple interpretations and readings, some of which may be in direct opposition to that which the creators intended (Miller et al. 1998, 210–11). This went beyond the immediate context of the campaign. In the mid-1990s, a 'look' became popular within the fashion world known as 'heroin chic'. Models displaying heroin chic had emaciated features with pale skin, dark circles underneath the eyes, and were often androgynous (Arnold 1999; Harold 1999; Hickman 2002). Visually, this look was similar to that portrayed in the Heroin Screws You Up campaign. Of course, the campaign did not lead directly to the creation of heroin

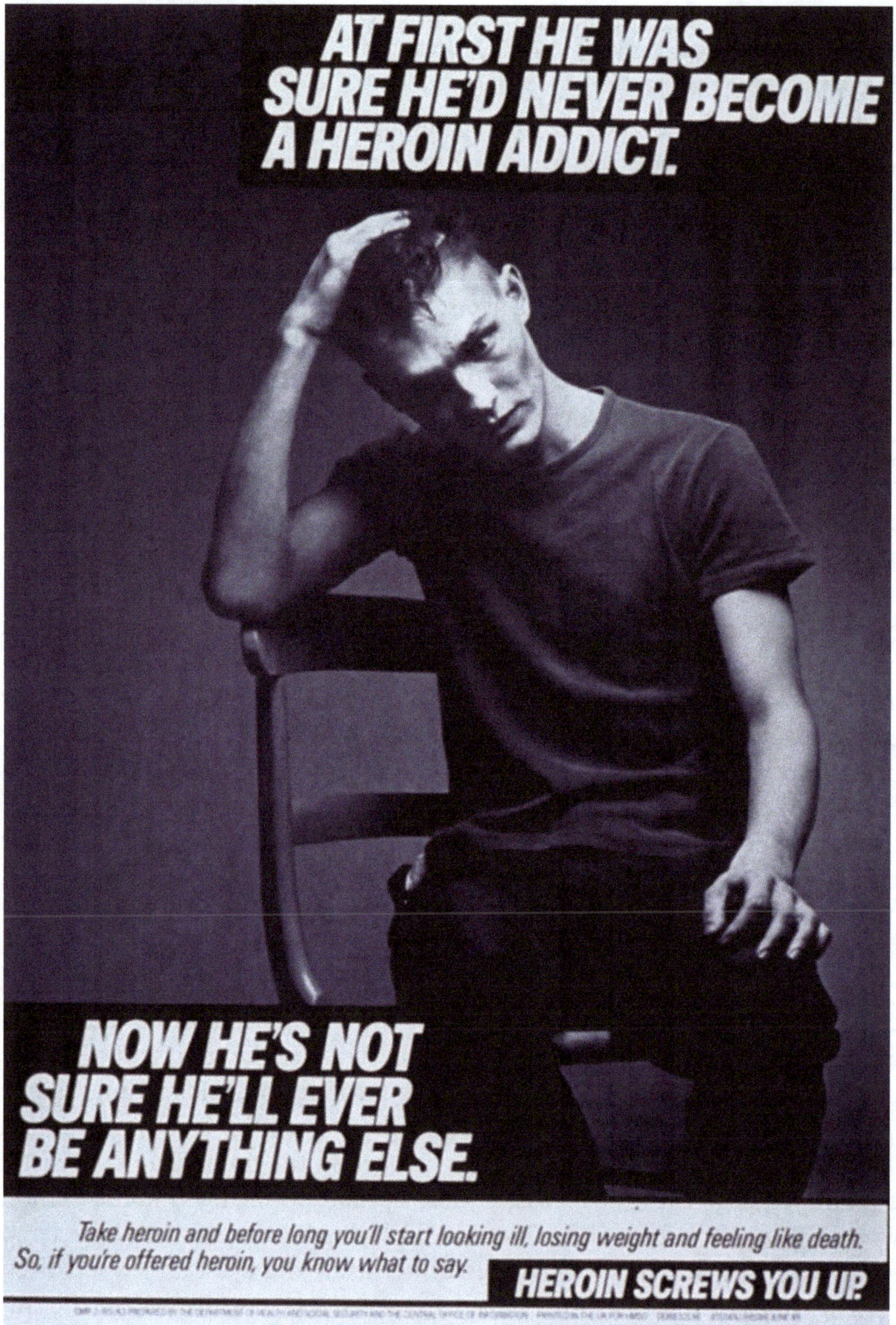
AT FIRST HE WAS
SURE HE'D NEVER BECOME
A HEROIN ADDICT.
NOW HE'S NOT
SURE HE'LL EVER
BE ANYTHING ELSE.
Take heroin and before long you'll start looking ill, losing weight and feeling like death.
So, if you're offered heroin, you know what to say.
HEROIN SCREWS YOU UP.

Fig. 4.1 Poster from the Heroin Screws You Up Campaign, 1985 (From the Department of Health and Social Security, Central Office of Information, shared under the Open Government licence. http://www.nationalarchives.gov.uk/doc/open-government-licence/version/3/)

chic. There were a whole host of other elements to this, but the similarity between the visuals, at least on the surface, speaks to the way in which imagery created for one purpose in one context is not owned by any one group or fit for one purpose. Just as the Heroin Screws You Up campaign drew on stereotypical images of drug users to try and sell an anti-drug message, the fashion industry could use similar visual tactics to sell clothes and a particular body image. The multiple readings and mobilisation of images was hardly unique to the 1980s, or to public health campaigns, but the enmeshing of motifs with commercial products illustrates the extent to which public health and its public had become embedded within the consumer society.

3.3 Lay Epidemiology

The influence of social and cultural context on the public's interpretation and reinterpretation of health education messaging was also at work in the development of the notion of 'lay epidemiology'. In evaluating 'Heartbeat Wales', a health promotion campaign aimed at informing the Welsh public about risk factors for cardiovascular disease, a group of epidemiologists and anthropologists coined a term to describe how the public interpreted those risks for themselves: 'lay epidemiology'. Their research participants, interviewed shortly after the miner's strikes of the early 1980s, constructed their beliefs about disease causation from a complex interaction between 'official' medical and public health sources, the mass media, and the lived experiences of friends, families and colleagues:

> [I]ndividuals interpret health risks through the routine observation and discussion of cases of illness and death in personal networks and in the public arena, as well as from formal and informal evidence arising from other sources, such as television and magazines. (Frankel et al. 1991)

Unlike in the previous decade, when the public had been largely absent or otherwise conceptualised as obliging receptacles for health education, in the 1980s that public also spoke back; or, at least, appeared to. The views, attitudes and beliefs of the public were a central concern of energetic and generously funded government campaigns such as 1987s 'Look After Your Heart' (LAYH), and the public responses to them.

Indeed, the LAYH campaign was to a certain extent predicated on the idea that many of the public were 'cynics' about the health education that they received. The newer era of market research driven health promotion campaigns ensured that ideas were audience tested and evaluated afterwards. LAYH was no different; the advertising agency Abbott Mead Vickers had run focus groups prior to creating television advertisements, while the Health Education Authority had commissioned Communication Research to conduct a survey on 'attitudes to heart disease' which found that 'people's general awareness of the causes and prevention of coronary heart disease is good' but 'that knowledge is not translated into action by nearly half of a representative sample of 1000 English adults' (Health Education Authority 1987a). LAYH's publicity materials were nothing if not gently self-deprecative; the explanatory text below a cartoon featuring the popular *Daily Mirror* character Andy Capp confided that:

> Being human, there is always a temptation to sit back and do nothing at all, and carry on the way you always have. Perhaps that's what Andy Capp would do. And perhaps the cheeky blighter would get away with and live to be 100. But there's a difference between Andy Capp and you. He is pen and ink. You are flesh and blood. (Health Education Authority 1987b, 11)

But if health education campaigns were attempting to incorporate the views and health beliefs of the public into their campaigns, it was those that sought to critique these campaigns that were most adept at harnessing voices of the public. Some public health professionals began using these dissenting views to more critically evaluate how public health communicated its messages. In a witness seminar on public health in the 1980s and 1990s, health services researcher Nick Black recollected that:

> there was a very exciting period in the early 1980s when public health was much more political ... One *samizdat* publication, by Wendy Farrant and Jill Russell ... couldn't be published, because it was an observational study by two sociologists of policy making in the Health Education Council on coronary heart disease prevention, where the policies were not informed by the evidence at all, actually completely counter to the evidence. They showed this with a lovely piece of qualitative research ... it got circulated among the younger, more radical public health folk. (Berridge et al. 2006, 40–41)

Black's use of the word '*samizdat*' [emphasis in the original] is instructive, pointing to both the apparently dissident nature of Farrant and Russell's work, and the views of the 'radical public health folk' on state-sponsored health education, allusive to the still-extant Soviet bloc. *The Politics of Health Information*, published in 1986 but possibly widely circulated before that, was deeply critical of current approaches (Health Education Authority 1990). While critical of HEC (and by extension its successor body, the Health Education Authority)'s attempts to '"sell" a "clear and simple" individualistic health education message' and its alleged selective use of epidemiological evidence, Farrant and Russell's most thrusting attack was that which was informed by their interviews with 21 informants (Farrant and Russell 1987, 39). Direct quotations were employed as ammunition to argue that the HEC's efforts were ineffectual and misguided. From these, we can see evidence of both a sceptical public, but also the manner in which this evidence was mobilised to make political points. Like those interviewed in Wales, respondents cited anecdotal and personal experiences that contradicted official narratives—'[t]here are people in their nineties who smoked all their lives, and are overweight, and as fit as a fiddle'—while also pointing to structural and socio-economic influences of people's lifestyles:

> [HEC] should also talk about the reasons why people eat bad diets and smoke – like the government's interest in perpetuating bad health by their interest in tax from tobacco sales. (Farrant and Russell 1987, 49, 54)

The dissident voices of the public were also broadcast by the media. In 1987, 'This Week's' TV documentary on heart disease and prevention programmes, *Lessons for the Living*, went into the pubs and social clubs of Sheffield to seek people's views on the city's attempts to address heart disease. Asking a young man whether he would be willing to change his lifestyle for a longer life, the presenter Jonathan Dimbleby received the reply, 'I go when I go, don't I?' The man's fatalism and indifference to the efforts of Sheffield's health education workers was used as a brickbat by the programme to denigrate current efforts. *Lessons for the Living* closed with the warning that 'unless more is done, Britain will continue to hold the worst record in the world' on combatting heart disease ('Lessons for the Living' 1987).

Despite attempts to integrate lay epidemiology into both the practice and critique of health promotion folk knowledge about heart disease remained resistant to official advice. Partly this was out of confusion about what constituted healthy living; as one middle-aged man on *Lessons for the Living* asked: 'Milk's no good for you, bread's no good for you, beer's no good for you, smoking's no good for you; what is good for us?' It was also born out of a feeling that life was brutish and short enough already; one widow told Farrant and Russell that '[m]y husband was on a 2000 calorie diet [before he died of heart disease] … salad—it takes all the pleasure out of living … better to live a shorter life' (Farrant and Russell 1987, 51). But perhaps the strongest explanation for this resistance was that of lived experience and the existence of a folk figure who illustrated a 'rich field of British cultural life, that of chance' which contradicted official epidemiological narratives (Davison et al. 1991, 14–15). This figure was:

> [a]n aged and healthy friend, acquaintance or relative – an "Uncle Norman" – who has smoked heavily for years, eats a diet rich in cream cakes and chips and/or drinks 'like a fish' is a real or imagined part of many social networks … A single Uncle Norman, it seems, may be worth an entire volume of medical statistics and several million pounds of official advertising. (Davison 1989, 46–47)

The public understanding of, and response to, public health campaigns was complex, nuanced and sometimes in direct opposition to the intended message. Health education campaigns and the images they produced did not exist in vacuum. Rather, these were part of a complex cycle of appropriation, reappropriation, interpretation and reinterpretation by the public.

4 Conclusion

Individuals were clearly capable of using the tools of public health, whether this be health education campaigns or the survey, to their own ends. This did not necessarily mean, however, that the long-running bargain between state and citizen over public health had tipped in favour of the individual. Many members of the public were aware that public health was concerned with collective health, and that this may involve some small element of personal sacrifice, whether that was the time spent talking to a surveyor or presenting one's child for vaccination. Yet, certain publics in certain contexts could resist such collective responsibilities in order to prioritise individual rights or personal preferences. As noted in Chapter 2, the broad narrative of health citizenship in the post-war period would suggest that over time the public became more concerned with individual rights and less interested in fulfilling collective duties. Our examples upset such a linear chronology. We found individuals refusing to participate in public health practices for their own reasons in the 1950s, just as most members of the public continued to accept a number of collective health responsibilities, such as vaccination. It is hard, perhaps impossible, to say if there was more 'speaking back' by the turn of the millennium than there had been in the middle of the century. As we discuss in Chapter 5, much of this revolves around the changing meaning of publicness and the forms which it took. Indeed, there is a need to move beyond seeing the public response to public health only in terms of rights and responsibilities. The public, we suggest, was capable of ascribing its own meaning or meanings to public health policies, practices and materials. The very nature of 'public', was, therefore, open to active reinterpretation.

Archival Material

Daily Mail, 2 August 1940, 8 November 1941; *Daily Express*, 27 July 1944, 3; 17 November 1949; *Sunday Express*, 11 June 1950; *The Times*, 30 June 1944, 5 February 1946, 10 December 1948.

HC Deb (27 April 1959) vol. 604, col. 880.

HC Deb (8 December 1989) vol. 163, cc. 581–638.

London School of Hygiene and Tropical Medicine (LSHTM) Archives: GB 0809 Whitehall/04/03/02: Correspondence regarding dietary habits postal survey.

LSHTM Archives, GB 0809 Whitehall/04/03/02: Correspondence regarding dietary habits postal survey, 21 January 1969.

LSHTM Archives, GB 0809 Whitehall/04/03/02: Correspondence regarding dietary habits postal survey, 26 January 1969.

LSHTM Archives, GB 0809 Whitehall/04/03/02: Correspondence regarding dietary habits postal survey, 3 June 1969.

LSHTM Archives, GB 0809 Whitehall/04/03/02: Correspondence regarding dietary habits postal survey, 15 July 1970.

Mass Observation at The Keep, SxMOA1/1/12/12/6, 15 "Anatomy of the 'Don't Knows,'" December 1947.

MOH for Stepney, Annual Report, 1950.

MOH for Surbiton, Annual Report, 1955.

MOH for Camberwell, Annual Report, 1959.

MOH for Woolwich, Annual Report, 1962.

TNA: MH 55/1745 correspondence and ephemera.

TNA: RG40/134: Complaints Received from Members of the Public Interviewed by S.S. Investigators, December 1949.

TNA: BN 10/229, A message from the Chief Medical Officer, December 1950.

TNA: MH 55/936, Diphtheria Prophylaxis: Publicity Campaign for Immunisation.

TNA: RG 40/133: Complaints Received from Members of the Public Interviewed by S.S. Investigators, 9 December 1947.

TNA: RG 40/134: Complaints Received from Members of the Public Interviewed by S.S. Investigators, 3 May 1951.

TNA: RG40/134: Complaints Received from Members of the Public Interviewed by S.S. Investigators, 8 May 1951.
TNA: RG 40/134: Complaints Received from Members of the Public Interviewed by S.S. Investigators, 9 May 1951.
TNA: RG40/134: Complaints Received from Members of the Public Interviewed by S.S. Investigators, 14 July 1951.
TNA: RG40/134: Complaints Received from Members of the Public Interviewed by S.S. Investigators, Fieldworker Report, 19 July 1950.
TNA: RG40/134: Complaints Received from Members of the Public Interviewed by S.S. Investigators, 21 July 1950.
TNA: RG 40/133: Complaints Received from Members of the Public Interviewed by S.S. Investigators, 29 November 1951.
TNA: RG 26/26: Survey of Sickness: Instructions to Interviewers.
TNA: RG 40/16: Health Index Survey: General Correspondence, 29 July 1948.
Wellcome Library: GC/178/A/2/4, Sidney Chave, Research Diary—The Health Survey, 6 May 1959.
Wellcome Library: GC/178/A/2/4, Sidney Chave, Research Diary—The Health Survey, 7 May 1959.
Wellcome Library: GC/178/A/2/4, Sidney Chave, Research Diary—The Health Survey, 22 May 1959.
Wellcome Library: GC/178/A/2/7, Sidney Chave, Research Diary—Collecting the GP Records, 4 January 1960.

Bibliography

Ahmed, Sara. n.d. 'Complaint'. *Feminist Killjoys Blog* (Blog). Accessed 6 June 2018. https://www.saranahmed.com/complaint/.

Arnold, Rebecca. 1999. 'Heroin Chic'. *Fashion Theory* 3 (3): 279–95.

Baggini, Julian. 2008. *Complaint: From Minor Moans to Principled Protests.* First Paperback edition. London: Profile Books.

Baker, Jeffrey P. 2003. 'The Pertussis Vaccine Controversy in Great Britain, 1974–1986'. *Vaccine* 21 (25–26): 4003–10.

Beers, Laura DuMond. 2006. 'Whose Opinion?: Changing Attitudes Towards Opinion Polling in British Politics, 1937–1964'. *Twentieth Century British History* 17 (2): 177–205.

Begg, Norman T., O. N. Gill, and Joanne M. White. 1989. 'COVER (Cover of Vaccination Evaluated Rapidly): Description of the England and Wales Scheme'. *Public Health* 103 (2): 81–89.

Berridge, Virginia. 2007. *Marketing Health: Smoking and the Discourse of Public Health in Britain, 1945–2000.* Oxford: Oxford University Press.

Berridge, Virginia, D. A. Christie, and E. M. Tansey, eds. 2006. *Public Health in the 1980s and 1990s: Decline and Rise.* London: Wellcome Trust.

Berridge, Virginia, Martin Gorsky, and Alex Mold. 2011. *Public Health in History.* 1st edition. Maidenhead: Open University Press.

Box, Kathleen, and Geoffrey Thomas. 1944. 'The Wartime Social Survey'. *Journal of the Royal Statistical Society* 107 (3/4): 151–89.

Cartwright, Ann. 1959. 'The Families and Individuals Who Did Not Cooperate on a Sample Survey'. *The Milbank Quarterly* 37 (4): 347–68.

Chen, Robert T., and Beth Hibbs. 1998. 'Vaccine Safety: Current and Future Challenges'. *Pediatric Annals* 27 (7): 445–55.

Clarke, John. 2014. 'Going Public: The Act of Complaining'. In *Complaints, Controversies and Grievances in Medicine*, edited by Jonathan Reinarz and Rebecca Wynter, 259–69. Oxford and New York: Routledge.

Colgrove, James Keith. 2006. *State of Immunity: The Politics of Vaccination in Twentieth-Century America.* Berkeley and New York: University of California Press and Milbank Memorial Fund.

Crook, Tom. 2016. *Governing Systems: Modernity and the Making of Public Health in England, 1830–1910.* Oakland: University of California Press.

Davison, Charlie. 1989. 'Eggs and Sceptical Eater'. *New Scientist* 1655: 45–49.

Davison, Charlie, George Davey Smith, and Stephen Frankel. 1991. 'Lay Epidemiology and the Prevention Paradox: The Implications of Coronary Candidacy for Health Education'. *Sociology of Health & Illness* 13 (1): 1–19.

Dobson, Roger. 2008. 'England and Wales Are Among European Countries at Highest Risk of Measles Epidemic'. *British Medical Journal* 336 (7635): 66–66.

Dohrenwend, Bruce P., and Barbara S. Dohrenwend. 1969. 'Sources of Refusals in Surveys'. *The Milbank Quarterly* 47 (1): 1153–54.

Douglas, John, and William Edgar. 1962. 'Smallpox in Bradford, 1962'. *British Medical Journal* 1 (5278): 612–14.

Durbach, Nadja. 2005. *Bodily Matters: The Anti-vaccination Movement in England, 1853–1907.* Durham, NC: Duke University Press.

Eriksen, Anne. 2016. 'Advocating Inoculation in the Eighteenth Century: Exemplarity and Quantification'. *Science in Context* 29 (2): 213–39.

Falk-Whynes, Jane. 1991. 'Drug Issues in Health Education: Demand Reduction of Public Panacea?' In *Policing and Prescribing: The British System of Drug Control*, edited by David Whynes and Philip Bean, 217–44. Basingstoke: Macmillan.

Farrant, Wendy, and Jill Russell. 1987. *The Politics of Health Information: 'Beating Heart Disease' as a Case Study of Health Education Council Publications.* London: University of London Institute of Education.

Fisher, Kate. 2008. *Birth Control, Sex, and Marriage in Britain 1918–1960.* Oxford: Oxford University Press.

Frankel, S., C. Davison, and G. D. Smith. 1991. 'Lay Epidemiology and the Rationality of Responses to Health Education'. *The British Journal of General Practice* 41 (351): 428–30.

Hansen, A. 1985. 'Will the Government's Mass Media Campaign on Drugs Work?' *British Medical Journal (Clinical Research Ed.)* 290 (6474): 1054–55.

Hargreaves, Ian, Justin Lewis, and Tammy Speers. 2003. *Towards a Better Map: Science, the Public and the Media*. London: Economic and Social Research Council.

Harold, Christine L. 1999. 'Tracking Heroin Chic: The Abject Body Reconfigures the Rational Argument'. *Argumentation and Advocacy* 36 (2): 65–76.

Health Education Authority. 1987a. *Attitudes to Heart Disease*. London: Health Education Authority.

———. 1987b. *Look After Your Heart: A Campaign to Encourage Healthier Lifestyles in England*. London: Health Education Authority.

———. 1990. *Beating Heart Disease*. London: Health Education Authority.

Heller, Jacob. 2008. *The Vaccine Narrative*. Nashville: Vanderbilt University Press.

Hickman, Timothy A. 2002. 'Heroin Chic: The Visual Culture of Narcotic Addiction'. *Third Text* 16 (2): 119–36.

Igo, Sarah E. 2009. *The Averaged American: Surveys, Citizens, and the Making of a Mass Public*. Cambridge, MA: Harvard University Press.

Larson, Heidi J., Caitlin Jarrett, Elisabeth Eckersberger, David M. D. Smith, and Pauline Paterson. 2014. 'Understanding Vaccine Hesitancy Around Vaccines and Vaccination from a Global Perspective: A Systematic Review of Published Literature, 2007–2012'. *Vaccine* 32 (19): 2150–59.

Larson, Heidi J., William S. Schulz, Joseph D. Tucker, and David M. D. Smith. 2015. 'Measuring Vaccine Confidence: Introducing a Global Vaccine Confidence Index'. *PLoS Currents Outbreaks* (February). https://doi.org/10.1371/currents.outbreaks.ce0f6177bc97332602a8e3fe7d7f7cc4.

'Lessons for the Living'. 1987. *Lessons for the Living*. ITV.

Lowy, Ilana. 2011. *A Woman's Disease: The History of Cervical Cancer*. Oxford: Oxford University Press.

Manning, Paul. 2013. '"No Reefer Madness Please—We're British": Accounting for the Remarkable Absence of Mediated Drugs Education in Post-war Britain 1945–1985'. *Media History* 19 (4): 479–95.

Marsh, Catherine. 1985. 'Informants, Respondents and Citizens'. In *Essays on the History of British Sociological Research*, edited by Martin Bulmer, 206–27. Cambridge: Cambridge University Press.

Marshall, T. H. 1992. 'Citizenship and Social Class'. In *Citizenship and Social Class*. London: Pluto Press.

Miller, David, Jenny Kitzinger, Kevin Williams, and Peter Beharrell, eds. 1998. *The Circuit of Mass Communication: Media Strategies, Representation and Audience Reception in the AIDS Crisis*. London: Sage.

Millward, Gareth. 2017a. '"A Matter of Commonsense": The Coventry Poliomyelitis Epidemic 1957 and the British Public'. *Contemporary British History* 31 (3): 1–23.

———. 2017b. 'A Disability Act? The Vaccine Damage Payments Act 1979 and the British Government's Response to the Pertussis Vaccine Scare'. *Social History of Medicine* 30 (2): 429–47.

Mitchell, Kirstin, Kaye Wellings, Gillian Elam, Bob Erens, Kevin Fenton, and Anne Johnson. 2007. 'How Can We Facilitate Reliable Reporting in Surveys of Sexual Behaviour? Evidence from Qualitative Research'. *Culture, Health & Sexuality* 9 (5): 519–31.

Mold, Alex. 2015. *Making the Patient-Consumer: Patient Organisations and Health Consumerism in Britain*. Manchester: Manchester University Press.

———. 2018. 'Exhibiting Good Health: Public Health Exhibitions in London, 1948–71'. *Medical History* 62 (1): 1–26.

Newlands, Emma. 2014. *Civilians into Soldiers: War, the Body and British Army Recruits, 1939–45*. 1st edition. Manchester and New York: Manchester University Press.

NHS. 2017. 'Childhood Vaccination Coverage Statistics, England, 2016–17', 20 September. https://digital.nhs.uk/data-and-information/publications/statistical/childhood-vaccination-coverage-statistics/childhood-vaccination-coverage-statistics-england-2016-17.

Power, Robert. 1989. 'Drugs and the Media: Prevention Campaigns and Television'. In *Drugs and British Society: Responses to a Social Problem in the 1980s*, edited by Susanne MacGregor, 129–42. London: Routledge.

Rafferty, Sarah, Matthew R. Smallman-Raynor, and Andrew D. Cliff. 2018. 'Variola Minor in England and Wales: The Geographical Course of a Smallpox Epidemic and the Impediments to Effective Disease Control, 1920–1935'. *Journal of Historical Geography* 59 (January): 2–14.

Research Bureau International. 1986. *Heroin Misuse Campaign Evaluation: Report of Findings*. London: Research Bureau International.

Rhodes, Tim. 1990. 'The Politics of Anti-drugs Campaigns'. *Druglink* (May/June): 16–18.

Robinson, Karen A., Cheryl R. Dennison, Dawn M. Wayman, Peter J. Pronovost, and Dale M. Needham. 2007. 'Systematic Review Identifies Number of Strategies Important for Retaining Study Participants'. *Journal of Clinical Epidemiology* 60 (8): 757–65.

Savage, Mike. 2010. *Identities and Social Change in Britain Since 1940: The Politics of Method*. Oxford and New York, NY: Oxford University Press.

Silcock, Jonathan, and Julie Ratcliffe. 1996. 'The 1990 GP Contract—Meeting Needs?' *Health Policy* 36 (2): 199–207.

Soazig, Clifton. 2014. 'Getting the Nation to Talk About Sex'. *Discover Society* (Blog), 6 January. https://discoversociety.org/2014/01/06/getting-the-nation-to-talk-about-sex/.

Taylor, Stephen James Lake Taylor, and Sidney Chave. 1964. *Mental Health and Environment*. Lond: Longmans.

Vincent, David. 2016. *Privacy: A Short History*. Cambridge, UK: Polity Press.

Wadsworth, M. E., S. L. Mann, B. Rodgers, D. J. Kuh, W. S. Hilder, and E. J. Yusuf. 1992. 'Loss and Representativeness in a 43 Year Follow Up of a National Birth Cohort'. *Journal of Epidemiology and Community Health* 46 (3): 300–304.

Wilson, Pixie, and Virginia Barker. 1944. *The Campaign Against Venereal Diseases*. London: COI.

Woodcock, Ruth. 1986. 'Would This Make You Stop and Think Twice?' *Health and Social Service Journal* (February 20): 248–49.

Yarwood, Joanne, Karen Noakes, Dorian Kennedy, Helen Campbell, and David Salisbury. 2005. 'Tracking Mothers Attitudes to Childhood Immunisation 1991–2001'. *Vaccine* 23 (48–49): 5670–87.

CHAPTER 5

Changing Publicness

Abstract In this chapter, we reflect not only on the challenges to publicness in public health but also its persistence. The increasing focus on individual behaviour as both a cause of disease and its remedy, posed a danger to collective understandings of the public and its health. Emphasising personal responsibility for health shifted liability from the state to the citizen, from public to private. At the same time, we point to ways in which publicness was retained, remade and even reinforced. 'The public' was increasingly recognised as an important actor in public health policy, practice and research. In the final section of the chapter, we consider developments beyond the dichotomy of 'public' and 'private' that were nonetheless crucial to changing conceptions of the public and public health.

Keywords Choice · Risk · Private · Public · Social structure · Environment

By now it should be abundantly clear that neither 'the public' nor 'public health' ever had a fixed or entirely coherent set of meanings. Yet, in the post-war period, the 'publicness' of public health seemed to undergo a radical shift. In this chapter, we reflect on both the challenges to publicness in public health but also its persistence. In the first section of the chapter, we concentrate on the increasing focus on individual behaviour as both a

A. Mold et al., *Placing the Public in Public Health in Post-War Britain, 1948–2012*, Medicine and Biomedical Sciences in Modern History,
https://doi.org/10.1007/978-3-030-18685-2_5

cause of disease and its remedy, and the ways in which this posed a danger to collective understandings of the public and its health. Emphasising personal responsibility for health shifted liability from the state to the citizen, from public to private. At the same time, in the second section of the chapter, we suggest that there were all sorts of ways in which publicness was retained, remade and even reinforced. 'The public' was increasingly recognised as an important actor in public health policy, practice and research. In the final section of the chapter, we consider developments beyond the dichotomy of 'public' and 'private' that were nonetheless crucial to changing conceptions of both the public, and public health policy and practice. Issues such as social structure and the environment impacted upon the public's health, but also influenced how people thought about the public. At the same time, new technologies offered fresh opportunities to create new public spaces and new publics.

Such complexity means we cannot tell a simple story of decline. The public has not 'fallen', but it has become penetrated by the private in a range of novel ways. The shifting boundaries of what could be considered public and what could be considered private, the making and remaking of various publics, and the spaces which they occupied, suggests that the public/private divide was increasingly hard to discern. Some might see this as private capture of the public sphere, but there were many ways in which the public, as a collection of people, as a space for action, and as a set of values, continued to matter. The blurring of boundaries between public and private health and the overlapping nature of publics and their interests may present problems of categorisation, but it did not signal the end of publicness in health.

1 Private

Interest in individual behaviour and the supposed 'privatisation' of public health were shifts peculiar to public health policy and practice, but they mirrored broader changes within British society and politics. From the late 1970s onwards in Britain, America and other high-income countries, neoliberal ideas began to influence many areas of government policy. Emphasis on individual entrepreneurial freedom, private property, free markets and free trade led to the development of policies that encouraged marketisation, privatisation and the prioritisation of individual wants and needs (Harvey 2007; Rodgers 2012). This led to the 'rolling back' of the state in the provision of public services. In healthcare, this was manifested most clearly in attempts to develop an internal market within the NHS and the growing use of private companies and private money to build hospitals and deliver services (Pollock 2005). Central to such 'neoliberal' (broadly defined) approaches was a view of the individual as sovereign. Individuals were thought to be best placed to make choices about their use of services, lives and interests (Le Grand 2007).

The influence of neoliberal ideas and policies paralleled changes in public health policy and practice in two areas. Firstly, in the growing emphasis on the individual, and secondly in the enhanced role for private companies within public health. Although public health policies and practices had intruded frequently into the private sphere, in the post-war period, the linking of chronic diseases to individual behaviour seemed to require a new level of interest in what had been private actions. In this section we consider how chronic disease prevention came to be reconfigured as a personal responsibility and a matter of individual choice. Such a shift was facilitated by the emergence of risk factor epidemiology that was able to calibrate an individual's risk of developing a specific condition. An increased focus on the individual was not, however, the only manifestation of 'the private' within public health. We also examine the growing role played by private companies in shaping the public's health.

1.1 *Personal Responsibility and Individual Choice*

Public health policymakers and practitioners had long been concerned with the private actions of individuals and the consequences these had for personal and collective health. Encouraging people to change their behaviour was a central part of early-twentieth-century health education efforts, but in the UK and in other high-income countries, the linking of lifestyle to disease from the 1950s onwards prompted closer interest in individuals and their conduct (Berlivet 2005; Rothstein 2003; Timmermann 2012; Fee and Acheson 1991). In Britain, the work of Richard Doll and Austin Bradford Hill on smoking and lung cancer was especially important in connecting individual behaviour to disease. In his classic text of 1957, the *Uses of Epidemiology*, Jerry Morris asserted that 'prevention of disease in the future is likely to be increasingly a matter of individual action and personal responsibility' (Morris 1957). As the list of behaviours that were thought to bring about ill-health expanded to encompass diet, exercise and alcohol, public health educators changed their approach to communicating with the public about threats to their health. For instance, the 1964 Cohen Report on health education recommended moving away from 'specific action campaigns', such as educating the public about vaccination, and towards areas of what it termed 'self-discipline', such as smoking, over-eating and exercise (Central Health Services Council and Scottish Health Services Council 1964).

By the mid-1970s, public health policy was increasingly orientated around the idea that individual behaviour was responsible for many public health problems. For example, in 1976, the government's major report on the public's health and how to improve it, *Prevention and Health, Everybody's Business*, asserted that:

> the weight of responsibility for his own health lies on the shoulders of the individual himself. The smoking related diseases, alcoholism and other drug dependencies, obesity and its consequences, and the sexually transmitted diseases are among the preventable problems of our time and in relation to all of these the individual must choose for himself. (Department of Health and Social Security 1976, 38)

Similarly, a few years later, in 1988, the Acheson report into the functioning of public health in England noted that:

> in recent years there has been a significant shift in emphasis in the perception of the determinants of the health of the public. In the context of the rise in importance of such conditions as cardiovascular disease and cancer, this now focusses far more than before on the effects of lifestyle and on the individual's ability to make choices which influence his or her own health. (Cm 289 1988, 2)

The role of public health authorities, was, according to public health practitioners John Ashton and Howard Seymour, to 'help make healthy choices the easy choices' (Ashton and Seymour 1988, 22). This could be achieved through regulation and legislative controls, but more often than not it was seen as the task of health education or health promotion.

As noted throughout the book, health education campaigns in the post-war period were frequently targeted at getting individuals to change their behaviour. Whether it was healthy eating, alcohol consumption or cigarette smoking, individuals were encouraged to take responsibility for their health by choosing an appropriate course of action (Hand 2017; Mold 2017; Berridge and Loughlin 2005). Such a view was predicated on a particular kind of self—an autonomous individual capable of self-government in response to expert advice (Miller and Rose 1990). People could choose to respond to illness or maintain their health within a broader culture of 'healthism' that situated the problem of sickness at the individual level (Armstrong 2009; Crawford 1980). As Deborah Lupton suggests, 'Healthism insists that the maintenance of good health is the responsibility of the individual, or the idea of one's health as an enterprise ... Healthism represents good health as a personal rational choice, "a domain of individual appropriation" rather than a vagary of fate' (Lupton 1995, 70). A focus on individual behaviour resulted in a conception of the public as a collection of self-governing rational actors able to respond to public health messages and change their behaviours accordingly. The role of the state, from a neoliberal perspective, was to facilitate the entrepreneurial actions of individuals rather than to create the broader social, economic and political conditions for good health (Ayo 2012). For Lupton, 'The concept of health as it is employed in contemporary public health and health promotion thus tends to individualise health and ill-health states, removing them from the broader social context' (Lupton 1995, 71). Under such logic, health, while not solely a private affair, was the prime responsibility of the individual not public authorities or actors. As we discuss in greater detail below, this view was not the only one in operation, but it was one that appeared to hold increasing appeal to governments of various political hues from the 1980s onwards.

1.2 Individual Risk

As discussed in Chapter 3, the emergence of risk-factor epidemiology and its comparison between the personal characteristics of groups to calculate probabilities of disease led to a focus on individual risk in the immediate post-war era. Nowhere was this more clearly articulated than by Morris, who noted that 'risks, chances and probabilities for the individual can be predicted, on average, from analysis of the collective experience of large numbers of representative individuals with the characteristics in question' (Morris 1957, 1955). These techniques, in part derived from the insurance industry, informed a 'new style of explaining cause and responsibility' in epidemiology, and, by extension, public health (Rothstein 2003; Aronowitz 2011; Giroux 2013).

The historian Dorothy Porter has used the figure of Morris as an avatar for post-war public health, arguing that *Uses of Epidemiology* provides evidence for Morris's declining interest in social class as an explanation for disease distribution, and that this 'allowed the deconstruction of the complexity of the social and biological relations of chronic diseases through the identification of "ways of living" as their primary cause'. From this, it followed that public health 'was able to offer the opportunity to prevent illness by changing social and individual behaviour' (Porter 2007, 82). Porter suggests that post-war public health authorities pursued 'a new hegemonic mission for preventive medicine that looked to reform personal and social behaviour rather than the reform of social structure as the route to a healthy society' (Porter 2002). While this individualisation of risk might have been most visible in exhortations for behaviour change, it was also evident in debates around the introduction of screening programmes for disease from the 1960s onwards. In some instances, this was a matter of the public themselves claiming the right to access the technologies of detecting as yet undiagnosed illness as a means of prevention, as with women's groups' campaigns for cervical cancer screening (Lowy 2011). For other diseases with multifactorial causes such as heart disease, however, some advocates viewed 'regular health examinations' as a potential means to provide tailored individual lifestyle advice to 'symptom-free individuals at high risk' (Turner and Ball 1973). However, the diagnostic accuracy of screening tests was a major barrier to such ambitions, with even contemporary comment in *The Lancet* conceding that:

> Identification of a susceptible individual has never really been achieved except through a gross averaged assessment of accumulated risk factors … a prediction within a high risk group on the basis of multiple factors still produces incorrect forecasts more often than correct ones. (Anon. 1974)

Indeed, debates on screening in the medical literature were largely predicated on technical issues of the sensitivity and specificity of any proposed tests, but resources were also considered an issue (Wilson and Junger 1968). Nonetheless, with the introduction of breast cancer screening in 1988, such programmes became an integral part of contemporary public health, with schemes addressing a wide number of cancers, maternal and new-born issues, as well as genetic conditions (Gov.uk, n.d.). In 2009, the NHS Health Check was introduced in England, with the objective of spotting early signs of stroke, kidney disease, heart disease, type 2 diabetes and dementia in adults aged 40–75, although take-up among the population was lower than anticipated (Clark et al. 2018). Although ascertaining and reducing individual risk of developing a chronic condition became crucial to public health practice, individuals themselves still needed to be persuaded of its benefits.

1.3 Private Companies and Public Health

An increased focus on individuals and their health was not the only way in which boundaries between public and private were redrawn in the post-war era. While in Porter's words, '[p]opulation health has always depended on collective provision of social welfare', private corporations began to take a significant interest in public health in Britain from the 1960s onwards (Porter 1999, 6). This interest took a number of forms, and was sometimes in partnership with state-based public health, and sometimes quite distinct from, and even in opposition, to it. Some companies used the research of epidemiology and discourse of public health education to help sell their products, while others sought to encourage their employees to practice healthier lifestyles. By the end of the twentieth century, some firms had even moved to providing established public health functions such as screening to their prospective customer base.

Historian Jane Hand has explored how Unilever, the 'leading food producer in post-war Britain', used emerging epidemiological evidence about the possible role of saturated fats in causing heart disease, and 'seized on societal reactions by engaging at-risk individuals as key agents of behavioural change, empowering them through consumption and the commodification of disease prevention' (Hand 2017, 482). Its advertising campaigns for Flora margarine targeted middle-aged men, as well as the housewives purportedly responsible for their husband's diet. For Hand, '[n]ot only were notions of "selling" health central to programmes of popular education at the behest of government but they also formed important components of marketing agendas by the food industry' (Hand 2017, 488). Indeed, in 2007 Unilever went further, offering blood cholesterol screening as part of its 'Test the Nation' campaign, using an established public health technique to market its product, conducting 72,000 tests and apparently adding £5.9m in sales value to Flora pro.activ (Unilever, n.d.).

As well as aligning themselves with public health discourses, corporate interests also sought to influence them. A snapshot of these efforts is provided by evidence given to a parliamentary inquiry into preventative medicine in the mid-1970s. While many witnesses who worked in public health had criticised elements of the food and tobacco industries, evidence provided by individuals representing such corporate interests demonstrated a more complicated and conflicted relationship between the two factions. For example, the Tobacco Research Council revealed that they continued to fund a number of epidemiological studies, including the Whitehall study of civil servants led by Donald Reid, who had given evidence to the inquiry on behalf of the London School of Hygiene and Tropical Medicine (Expenditure Committee 1977, 805). Alongside providing funding for such research activities, corporations were also keen to use epidemiological data to bolster their own arguments regarding prevention, especially when it might dovetail with the promotion of their products. The manufacturer of Flora margarine repeatedly lobbied the inquiry and government ministers to endorse poly-unsaturated fats, as well as noting that Jerry Morris, in giving evidence, had mentioned its product by name (GI Grant, letter to A Milner-Barry, n.d.). Other food industry bodies such as the National Dairy Council highlighted uncertainty in the research literature to try to prevent the committee forming adverse opinions about milk, butter and their potential link to Coronary Heart Disease (CHD) (National Dairy Council 1976). Finally, the John Lewis Partnership highlighted the preventative work they were conducting with their employees, offering screening for cardiovascular disease and fitness campaigns for staff, a model that would be adopted as part of the 'Look After Your Heart' campaign in the 1980s (WM Dixon, letter to A Milner-Barry, 2 January 1976). The boundary between 'private' companies and 'public' health efforts, was therefore, increasingly blurred.

2 Public

Despite the increased focus on private actions and private companies with public health, there were also a number of ways in which publicness was retained and even strengthened. Just as neoliberalism was unable to entirely erode social democracy in other sectors of British politics and society, large parts of what was thought of as related to 'public health' remained 'public' (Vernon 2017, 476–516). This can be seen in the extent to which 'the public' and its needs became a topic of both political and research interest. In this section, we consider how calls for increased public representation in healthcare impacted upon public health policy and practice. We also look at how social scientists attempted to create a picture of the health of the whole public through the development of the concept of 'population' and the representative survey.

2.1 Representation

From the 1960s onwards, there was increasing pressure for greater public representation within healthcare in Britain. Some of this momentum came from patients and the public (Mold 2013). Patient organisations and other voluntary groups demanded a say in their own treatment and the shape and direction of health services. By the 1970s, the government recognised that there was a need to take patient and public views into account. Following the reorganisation of the NHS in 1973 Community Health Councils (CHCs) were set up in every local health authority in England (similar mechanisms were put in place for Scotland, Wales and Northern Ireland). These were intended to be the 'voice of the consumer' within the NHS (Joseph 1973). Although the CHCs were highly variable in their effectiveness, they did provide a means through which public views on health services (including public health) could be heard (Mold 2015, 42–68; Hogg 2009). During the 1980s, the number of organisations claiming to represent the opinions and needs of patients and the public in health grew considerably (Salter 2003; Wood 2000; Baggott et al. 2005). At the same time, the figure of the patient, and particularly the 'patient-consumer' grew in political saliency as first the Thatcher, and then Major governments made substantial changes to the organisation of the NHS. The introduction of the internal market in 1989 and the establishment of the *Patient's Charter* in 1991, were supposed to give patients greater rights within a more consumer-orientated service (Mold 2012, 2015, 94–116). Although the precise mechanisms for achieving patient and public representation within healthcare changed frequently following the scrapping of the CHCs in 2003, the imperative for such representation did not go away. An 'alphabet soup' of organisations were created to provide public representation in health, although questions can be raised about their effectiveness (Forster and Gabe 2008; Hogg 2009; Baggott 2005). At the same time, representation often focused on healthcare and the NHS, rather than public health or public health services per se (Baggott and Jones 2011). Indeed, public representation within public health services and practices and was especially difficult. In part, this was a result of the changing position of public health services within the health system, but also because it was difficult to provide opportunities for representation across a wide range of services, issues and areas.

That does not mean, however, that the public went unrepresented within public health. One way in which this was achieved was through health surveys. Surveys were a technology through which public needs could be shaped and represented by public health authorities, but they could also act as an arena for the articulation of certain needs by different publics, providing evidence to support demands. In the late 1960s, the Department of Health and Social Security (DHSS) commissioned a survey from the Government Social Survey (GSS) department on the experiences of the 'chronic sick and physically handicapped' living in Britain. This survey aimed to chart the numbers of people in Britain living with disability or chronic illness and the effects their conditions had on their lives. The DHSS intended to use the information gathered in the survey to shape its policy decisions regarding the benefits made available to disabled people.

In rethinking the provision of services available to disabled people, the DHSS was not operating in a vacuum. In 1965, the publication of Peter Townsend and Brian Abel-Smith's *The Poor and the Poorest* represented the high point of a 'rediscovery of poverty' in Britain that had been building from the late-1950s onwards (Hampton 2016). As it became clear that the welfare state had not eradicated poverty, especially in neglected demographics such as elderly and disabled people, a 'poverty lobby' emerged composed of voluntary organisations which campaigned on behalf of these disadvantaged sections of society (Oliver and Campbell 1996; Whitely and Winyard 1987). This included organisations such as the Disablement Income Group (DIG) which was also established in 1965. DIG was the first advocacy group formed and led by disabled people. It was set up by two disabled housewives in Godalming, Surrey, after they wrote a letter to the *Guardian* women's page (Stott 1989, 77; Hilton et al. 2013, 61). Initially formed to highlight the difficulties of disabled women, DIG campaigned for a non-contributory 'National Disability Income' for all disabled people based on need (Millward 2015, 275–76; Hampton 2016, 88). The DHSS was very conscious of the political climate surrounding its investigations into disabled people's lives and needs. A draft paper from the Ministry of Social Security in spring 1968 wrote of the 'considerable volume of complaint about the present arrangements' and noted the 'sustained and heavy pressure ... exerted' by 'the Disablement Income Group ... the National Council for the Single Woman, the National Campaign for the Young Chronic Sick, the Press, and Members of Parliament of all Parties' (DHSS, Proposed Survey of the number and needs of chronic sick and handicapped people, 1968).

Although the survey was largely developed by the GSS in conference with the DHSS and Margot Jefferys from Bedford College, the DHSS also consulted DIG (Harris 1971). DIG was given a draft copy of the questionnaire, and asked to provide evidence and advice based on a recognition that it had a 'unique expertise … in knowing where disabled people lived and what questions might be pertinent to the issues they faced' (Millward 2015, 284). Although the 'public' nature of DIG is somewhat contested—the group's patrons included senior academics and politicians, and from 1969 onwards their leaders were well-educated and included ex-civil servants—this was a case of public pressure being exerted on the Government in a moment of reform (Millward 2015, 278). Through campaigning, DIG's expertise was recognised, and they were able to shape the Government's research to make sure the survey asked questions which articulated their needs and those of other disabled people in Britain. The survey findings were later used in the development of an Attendance Allowance, Invalidity Benefit, and the 1975 Social Security Benefits Act which created benefits of disabled housewives (Millward 2015, 280). In this way, a disabled public contributed to its remaking through the mechanism of the public health survey.

Although 'the public' was increasingly recognised as an important actor in public health research, not all publics were recognised in the same way or given the same platform. By the 1980s, people of colour were utilising the survey to fight against health inequalities and discrimination, and to draw attention to issues they felt were otherwise left off the agenda of public health. One example of this was Elizabeth Anionwu and Usha Prashar's research into screening and counselling facilities for sickle cell anaemia which found services to be lacking and raised the issue of racial discrimination. In *Sickle Cell Anaemia: Who Cares?* Anionwu and Prashar wrote of an indifferent public health service. They suggested that sickle cell disorders had been seen as 'rare tropical illness and of little significance in Britain', with the consequence that health officials received little information about them in their training (Prashar and Anionwu 1985, 8). Although the Organisation for Sickle Cell Research (1975) and the Sickle Cell Society (1979) 'constantly attempted to highlight the problems facing' those with sickle cell disorders (SCD), Anionwu and Prashar argued that little had been done by public health. Sponsored by the Runnymede Trust, their survey investigated what services were available to SCD patients within the NHS. The survey found that services were 'ad hoc and patchy' with 'no central guidelines and … no resources … made available either centrally or locally' (Prashar and Anionwu 1985, 50). SCD had been left out of the 1975 NHS Resource Allocation Working Party (an attempt to redistribute resources within the NHS) formula (Gorsky and Millward 2018).

Anionwu and Prashar used these findings to argue that funds should be 'allocated centrally for the development of comprehensive care for SCD and that firm guidelines [be] issued on the principles, aims and structures of such care' (Prashar and Anionwu 1985, 51). Following this, Anionwu's Ph.D. research explored health education and community action around sickle cell anaemia in the London borough of Brent and brought to the fore the 'harrowing experiences' of BME parents she surveyed whose children had been diagnosed with it. Despite her focus, Anionwu wrote that it was:

> vital to stress that this thesis is not advocating that black health workers restrict themselves to specific conditions relevant to black people. Singling out particular conditions for attention, such as SCD or rickets has rightly been condemned in various quarters as providing an opportunity for health authorities to side-track the most important issue, that of institutional racism. (Anionwu 1988)

Anionwu continued to centre the effects of racism, institutional and otherwise, on the health and healthcare of people of colour in Britain in her work. Later she advocated for a national register for SCD, suggesting that more accurate information regarding the estimated national prevalence of the condition might strengthen the case for support (Anionwu and Atkin 2001, 2, 121). In this way, when government-led research was not forthcoming, publics created and called for surveys of their own to support demands for services which they considered neglected by public health.

2.2 Population

The survey was not just a tool for specific publics to get their needs onto the agenda. Public health authorities' expansion and interpretation of statistics, including the use of the representative survey, played a vital role in determining how population health was viewed by policymakers and what actions should be taken to improve it (Szreter 2002). A new, more comprehensive conception of the public as objects of, and participants in, research and the governance of health began to take hold (Crook 2016, 295). At the heart of the representative survey is the notion that 'the part can replace the whole', but, as Alain Desrosières suggests, the idea of representativeness forces the questions: 'What is part? What is whole?', and in turn demands definition of the population, or 'whole public', in which the two are firmly linked (Desrosières 2010). In post-war Britain, through surveys and representative sampling, public health consistently used parts of the public to represent the whole population. But the questions asked of these representative members of the public and the categories they were subsequently sorted into changed, thus altering the conception of the 'whole public' as well as reflecting a public that had also changed.

The clearest example of this can be seen in Britain's whole-population birth cohort studies, starting with the National Survey of Health and Development in 1946, and followed successively by the National Childhood Development Study in 1958, the 1970 British Birth Cohort Study, and the UK Millennium Cohort Study in 2000. In 1946, the National Survey of Health and Development questionnaire asked 'mothers' to categorise themselves through questions about size of the household and occupation of the baby's father (Royal College of Obstetricians and Gynaecologists and the Population Investigation Committee 1946). Of the initial 13,687 responses to the maternity survey, 5362 children were sampled for follow-up including 'all single births to married women with husbands in non-manual and agricultural employment and 1 in 4 of all comparable births to women with husbands in manual employment' (Wadsworth et al. 2006). In the 1958 and 1970 studies, all survivors from the original sample of all babies born in the study week were selected to remain in the study, including those born to unmarried women (Power and Elliott 2006). The 1958 and 1970 questionnaires each asked the participant mothers about their husband's occupation, and their own work before pregnancy, though the 1970 questionnaire afforded these equal weight, whereas the 1958 version positioned the mother's work as more of an afterthought (Centre for Longditudinal Studies, n.d.). Like the 1946 study, the 1958 National Child Development Study Birth Cohort did not ask its participant mothers for their ethnicity. The 1970 British Birth Cohort Study's first survey also contained no questions about ethnicity. By 2000, however, the Millennium Cohort sample was constructed to be 'representative of the total UK population', but 'certain sub-groups of the population were intentionally over-sampled, namely children living in disadvantaged areas, children of ethnic minority backgrounds and children growing up in the smaller nations of the UK'. The disproportionate representation of these groups was to ensure that 'typically hard to reach populations' were 'adequately represented' and that sample sizes were 'sufficient for ... analysis' (Connelly and Platt 2014). Study members were asked a much broader range of questions than previous surveys: 'Are you married to the baby's father/ separated/ divorced/ just friends/ not in any relationship?', 'How many hours of child care do you pay for each week?', 'Did you have any medical fertility treatment for this pregnancy?' (Pearson 2016; Centre for Longditudinal Studies, n.d.) While these questions reflected changes to lifestyle, and changes in the interest of the surveyors, they were ultimately facilitated by new technology: questionnaires were completed on computers. A greater number of questions could be included than on cumbersome paper schedules, and the data gathered could be more easily organised (Pearson 2016, 264).

Neither the 1946 study nor the 2000 study encompassed a 'whole public' physically living in Britain, instead their study population selections reflected the continuities and changes present in the interests of the public health surveyors, albeit with carefully 'adjusted analyses to provide accurate prevalence estimates and robust standard errors' (Connelly and Platt 2014, 1719). In 1946, the concern of the Population Investigation Committee-commissioned study was over British birth rates, and this was reflected in the sampling of white British children born to married parents (Pearson 2016, 19). In 2000, the surveyors were still driven to understand how disadvantage in early life affected health and development in later years, hence the over-sampling of children living in poverty, but they had a new interest in Britain's growing minority ethnic population, and so over-sampled children from those backgrounds as well (Pearson 2016, 261). As Desrosières suggests, although these statistical methods were originally developed by eugenicists, what is remarkable is that the 'techniques quickly became … almost obligatory checkpoints for proponents of other views'. Statistics continued to 'structure … the very terms of debates, and the language spoken in the space of the politico-scientific debate' (Desrosières 2010, 329). As such, the 'whole public' represented through public health surveys tended to reflect the parts of the whole which were of particular interest to the surveyors and to public health, while also mirroring changes in society.

Some of the tensions between the individual and their relation to the wider population were explored in the late 1980s by Geoffrey Rose, a researcher on the Whitehall studies, but also a vastly experienced and well-respected figure in epidemiological circles internationally. His seminal paper 'Sick individuals, sick populations' was a key intervention at a time when questions were being asked about the role of prevention, health education and health promotion. While in the 1970s there had been a widespread consensus on the principle of prevention, by the middle of the 1980s this had splintered. Rose clarified many of the conceptual issues, using examples from his own research. Firstly, he outlined how epidemiologists were able to find out which individuals were at high risk of disease, by examining their differential exposures to a particular risk factor. But if that risk factor were common—for example, if everybody smoked twenty cigarettes a day—then it would be very difficult to work out what that risk factor or behaviour was, because everyone's exposure would be the same, and incidence of disease would only vary based on individual genetic susceptibility. The epidemiologist would instead have to turn to comparing different populations—for example, British civil servants and Kenyan nomads—who had entirely different rates of the same disease and work out what exposure was common in one group but not in the other (Rose 1985).

While on its own this might seem the type of insight that could appear in an epidemiology textbook, Rose argued that this had much wider implications about societal disease prevention. His view was that up until this point, public health policy had been too fixated on the identification of 'high-risk' groups. While this approach had its merits (and he pointed to the relative success of the smoking cessation randomised controlled trial in Whitehall I), and could potentially be very motivational for the individuals concerned, Rose identified some problems, which he argued were particularly salient for a 'mass disease' like CHD. Firstly, that any screening programme would inevitably miss 'borderline' cases who might have also benefited from whatever intervention was available. Secondly, and more significantly:

> [screening] is palliative and temporary, not radical. It does not seek to alter the underlying causes of the disease but to identify individuals who are particularly susceptible to those causes ... it does not deal with the root of the problem, but seeks to protect those who are vulnerable to it; and they will always be around. (Rose 1985, 36)

Rose insisted that this problem was particularly acute for heart disease, Britain's biggest killer. Because it was so common in such post-industrial countries, it was difficult for screening to discriminate between low and high-risk individuals. Rose personalised this dilemma:

> I have long congratulated myself on my low levels of coronary risk factors ... [t]he painful truth is that for such an individual in a Western population the commonest cause of death – by far – is coronary heart disease! Everyone, in fact, is a high-risk individual for this uniquely mass disease. (Rose 1985, 37)

The implications of this could be read in two ways. On the one hand, it could be argued that prevention was 'everybody's business', as the government green paper had suggested a decade earlier (Department of Health and Social Security 1976). However, Rose was sceptical about highlighting individual responsibility for disease prevention, arguing that '[e]ating, smoking, exercise and all our other life-style characteristics are constrained by social norms'. Public health should therefore be concentrating on shifting social norms, or better still, 'remov[ing] the underlying causes that make the disease common' (Rose 1985, 37). Nonetheless, Rose acknowledged that prevention at the population level had some drawbacks, the most problematic of which was the 'prevention paradox'. This he summarised as a 'preventative measure which brings much benefit to the population offers little to each participating individual', a predicament that he claimed had been 'the history of public health – of immunization, the wearing of seat belts and now the attempt to change various life-style characteristics' (Rose 1985, 38).

Rose's unsparing appraisal of the contradictions of lifestyle public health and its focus on the individual was his 'big idea' (Hofman and Vandenbroucke 1992). It used insights from the Whitehall study to reason that trying to change people's behaviour without changing the circumstances in which they practice that behaviour was at best only ever going to be partially successful. In his later book, *The Strategy of Preventive Medicine*, Rose expanded this critique to get to the core of how he thought public health should view itself:

> in order to grasp the principles of public health one must understand that society is not merely a group of individuals but is also a collectivity ... Society is important in public health because it profoundly effects the lives and thus the health of individuals. (Rose 1992)

Over the next two decades Rose's idea would be endlessly debated, critiqued and celebrated in epidemiological and medical journals (Charlton 1995; Færgeman 2005; Doyle et al. 2006). He was successful in prompting a fundamental questioning of the tenets of the prevailing paradigm of lifestyle public health. Using his experience from the first Whitehall study, Rose had argued that focussing on the individual's susceptibility to a risk factor was only half the story; public health had also to consider the risk factor itself. Furthermore, the way in which society promulgated norms, and indeed organised itself, had health effects for individuals. There was, then, no simple divide between public actions with private health effects, or private actions with public health effects.

3 Beyond Public and Private

In the post-war period there were a number of important shifts that had a significant impact on public health that could not be easily categorised as either 'public' or 'private'. The complex relationship between social structure, and especially social inequality, in health outcomes illustrates the interaction between public and private in shaping individual and collective health. Moreover, as we discuss in this section, there were other factors that also played a role in determining population health, such as the environment. Towards the end of our period, novel technologies offered new possibilities for re-imaging the public or publics and their health. Seeing beyond the public/private divide allows us to rethink both.

3.1 Social Structure

Writing in *The Lancet* in 1986, Alex Scott-Samuel, a public health doctor in Liverpool, argued that 'social inequalities in health [were] back on the agenda' (Scott-Samuel 1986). In part a concise summary of the depth and breadth of health inequalities research that the 1980 Black Report had sparked, it also pointed to the impression that up to this point, structural and socioeconomic determinants of health had been somewhat neglected as public health policy pursued an individualistic lifestyle agenda in post-war Britain. While some commentators have challenged this view, there can be no doubt that the 1980s saw a resurgence of research interest into differentials in health (Macintyre 2002). Scott-Samuel's article noted 'the number of "local Black reports" by both statutory and community agencies' that had been produced, as well as placing the Whitehall I research alongside recent work by sociologists and social policy researchers such as Mildred Blaxter, Julian Le Grand and David Blane. Blaxter's research primarily concerned health service use and the intergenerational effects of poverty and inequality, while Le Grand wrote extensively on structural and fiscal explanations for inequality (Blaxter 1983; Blaxter and Paterson 1982; Le Grand 1978; Muurinen and Le Grand 1985). Both offered correctives to suggestions that disparities in health were either a product of people's lifestyles, or merely a matter of statistical artefact. Blane focused on the Black Report as a means to address some of the main criticisms that had been levelled at health inequalities research. His analysis identified four principle explanations for the disparities that Black had identified: artefact; selection; cultural or behavioural; and materialist (Blane 1985).

The artefactual critique referred to the possibility that the way in which the five social classes had been defined by the Registrar General since 1913 might firstly be too crude to accurately describe the complexities of class and its relation to occupation, and secondly, that 'the workforce in semi and unskilled manual jobs is shrinking as such work is increasingly mechanised and automated … newer [younger] recruits to the workforce must move into skilled or white-collar jobs' (Blane 1985, 424). The consequence of this was that disparities in mortality would be exaggerated because older people would be overrepresented in lower social classes. While this explanation could be relatively easily eliminated by adjusting for age in statistical models, Blane also cited Whitehall I as being instrumental in rejecting this explanation, as the clearer hierarchical divisions present in an otherwise 'homogenous industry' than in society at large meant that rank in itself was plainly a factor.

The narrative of selection posited that healthier people were likely to move up the social classes. Critics suggested that health inequalities research had been too static in its analysis, failing to take into consideration the longitudinal effects of social mobility. Indeed, this critique stretched back to the 1950s and the sociologist Raymond Illsley's work on infant mortality (Illsley 1955; Stern 1983). Blane conceded that selection might well be a 'real phenomenon … [but] data suggest that it is small, and that even this is limited to certain age groups and parts of the social structure' (Blane 1985, 431). The Whitehall researchers had also been alive to this issue; Michael Marmot had lamented privately that 'when examining the relationship of grade to mortality in the original Whitehall Study, we had no information on job histories' (M Marmot to AM Semmence, 7 August 1980). Whitehall II attempted to address this by maintaining regular contact with the civil servants, and asking questions about their employment history to provide a more rounded picture of how they might move up or down hierarchies. Ultimately, Blane was insistent that '[o]nly materialist explanations can simultaneously account for both … the improvement in general health and the maintenance of class differences in health' observed in post-war Britain. Importantly, he argued that lifestyle explanations could also be subsumed into this analysis, again citing papers from the first Whitehall study to bolster his arguments. Individuals made choices constructed by their socioeconomic circumstances: 'behaviour cannot be separated from its context' (Blane 1985, 434).

Blane's assessment of the Black Report provides a snapshot of several of the key issues in health inequalities research during its boon in the 1980s. His analysis of the evidently contested nature of health inequalities research, and the theoretical challenges directed at it, prefigured the controversy that would engulf Margaret Whitehead's *The Health Divide*, published in 1987 and widely viewed as the follow-up to the Black Report (Townsend et al. 1982; Berridge 2002). Blane's recollections elsewhere of his experiences in the early 1980s also reveal the tight professional and educational links between many of these researchers (Blane 1985, 16). Similarly, John Fox, a statistician whose work contributed to the Black Report, recalled that:

> I think that there was more research done in the 1980s on health inequalities than at any other time ... [there] was a background for lots of people supporting each other, strong networks building up, which didn't exist before that time. (Berridge 2002, 168)

The flame of health inequalities research continued to be carried throughout the 1990s most prominently by the Whitehall II study, which reported in 1991 that their 'findings show[ed] that socioeconomic differences in health status have persisted over the 20 years separating the two Whitehall studies' (Marmot et al. 1991). From this juncture onwards, the Whitehall studies began to become a byword for health inequalities in public discourse. Michael Marmot cannily used evidence from Whitehall in the publication of the Acheson Report on health inequalities in 1998, and would lead his own review of the issue in 2010 (Acheson 1998; Marmot 2010). In recent years, popular books from Richard Wilkinson and Kate Pickett, social geographer Danny Dorling and economist Joseph E. Stiglitz have also helped to highlight the issue to politicians and policymakers (Pickett and Wilkinson 2010; Dorling et al. 2015; Stiglitz 2013) to the extent that ahead of the 2010 election then Conservative leader of the opposition David Cameron ambitiously (if ultimately fallaciously) promised to 'banish health inequalities to the history books', arguing they were one of the 'most unjust, unfair and frankly shocking things about life in Britain today' (Bowcott 2010).

3.2 *The Environment*

Health inequalities were, of course, not a new factor in influencing collective health, and other, older, factors such as the environment, also had an enduring legacy. Notions of the environment were central to nineteenth-century public health practice, but in the middle part of the twentieth century, as public health's gaze turned towards the individual, the perceived influence of space and place on health altered. Some, more traditionally 'environmental' concerns did persist. Medical Officers of Health, for example, retained their role in policing environmental health, a responsibility they took seriously (Jackson 2005; Thorsheim 2009; Corton 2015). During the 1950s, air pollution posed a particular threat to public health. The burning of coal significantly reduced air quality, and in 1952, the Great Smog led to thousands of deaths, especially in London (Berridge and Taylor 2005). As a result, the Clean Air Act was introduced in 1956. The Act required those living in smoke control areas to burn smokeless fuels in their homes (Berridge and Gorsky 2012). Yet, in some ways, air pollution was the exception that proved the rule: the environment mattered as a political issue, but it was seen as a separate topic, one that had little to do with public health (Berridge 2007, 208). For Berridge, 'The environment had been almost entirely absent from the redefined public health ideology that had emerged in the 1970s … New concerns about occupational health or about environmental pollution had no particular connections with public health' (Berridge 2007, 208).

Yet, by the 1980s, there were signs of a different understanding of the environment and its impact on health. David Armstrong argues that the environment was seen as posing two kinds of threat. The first concerned the interaction of bodies with nature including new environmental dangers such as 'noxious gases from car exhausts in the air; chemicals from aerosols in the ozone layer; acid rain from industry in the water and pollution in the soil …'. The second concerned the dangers that bodies themselves posed, or more accurately the behaviours of particular bodies. The AIDS epidemic, Armstrong asserts, existed 'within a context of wider social activities: at one level the problem is conceptualised in terms of the socialising patterns or culture of gay men; at another it is the complex social interactions involved in needle sharing and blood transfusion' (Armstrong 1993, 405). The revival of infectious disease as a public health issue in the form of HIV/AIDS, as Berridge also points out, required public health policymakers and practitioners to reconsider the role of the environment. Indeed, the environment came to be seen as crucial not just to the aetiology of communicable disease, but to chronic disease too. Passive smoking, for example, brought together a concern for their individual and their behaviour with the physical environment and the generation of second-hand smoke (Berridge 2007, 208–40). By the late 1990s, the conceptualisation of the 'environment' and its impact on the public's health appeared to have widened still further. Public health issues such as obesity were increasingly depicted in environmental terms. The notion of the 'obesogenic environment', or the response of normal physiology to an abnormal environment, relied upon a notion of the environment that is both physical, but also economic and sociocultural (Egger and Swinburn 1997). In some ways, then, 'the environment' has come to be a synonym for the structural influences on the public's health, but one that places emphasis not just on socioeconomic structure, but on space and place too.

3.3 New Spaces

Changes in information and communication technology in the last decades of the twentieth century created new spaces that allowed for new forms of interaction between publics and public health authorities. One of the most radical changes in communication in recent years is the arrival of the World Wide Web. Although publicly released in 1993, it was not until the turn of the millennium that this technology became widely accessible to British people (UNdata, n.d.). Nevertheless, as usage increased, public health authorities had to grapple with the speed and volume of communication that was now possible. 'The internet'—as a technology, an information store and the cultures built around its use—was a new space for the making and remaking of both the public and private spheres and associated actors, something historians are beginning to get to grips with (Abbate 2017; Turner 2017). Although the internet only appeared towards the end of our period, it was already becoming crucial in assessing what the public was, how it expressed itself and how it was understood by public health authorities.

One of the most prominent ways in which the internet figured in recent debates about public health was during the crisis around the Measles Mumps and Rubella (MMR) vaccine (c. 1998–2004) (Speers and Lewis 2004). Anti-vaccination and MMR-sceptic information was shared through static web pages online, but there is clear evidence that parents with internet access were sharing this information with others in their peer group

(Selway 1998). Such interactions demonstrated that many General Practitioners were not vaccination experts, and so were unable to adequately counter detailed and specific complaints about vaccinology, epidemiology and alternatives to the triple-dose vaccine (Petrovic et al. 2001). Parents also expressed uncertainty as a result of being presented contradictory information from doctors, the government, the press, fellow parents and the internet. In response, the Department of Health made a concerted effort to use this new technology to educate both parents *and* health professionals about the importance of MMR to the public's health in 2002. Utilising recent developments in risk communication tools, the website 'MMR: The Facts' and specific guidance issued through the Department of Health's webpages for health professionals directly answered the 'myths' and counter-arguments offered by vaccine sceptic groups (Department of Health 2002a, b). The internet thus offered an outlet for non-traditional voices to express concerns and challenge expertise, but it was also a forum for expertise to speak back to its critics and tailor its responses to those publics most susceptible to these counter narratives.

As internet usage increased, other sources of public behaviour and interaction with the internet beyond vaccination should be considered. The traditional press, often in a mocking tone, highlighted the public's use of websites such as *WebMD* to self-diagnose and suggested that this might be exacerbating latent hypochondria in the population (Baxter 2013). Similarly, the cultural reception of *MumsNet*, a community predominantly of mothers sharing parenting advice, questions and frustrations, tells us much about attitudes towards motherhood. The site itself, however, could be a rich vein of data about the sorts of health issues parents were concerned about over time, since it includes not just edited blog posts but also forum contributions and responses from mothers themselves. These have been articulated and preserved in a way that few pre-internet age sources can provide.

Finally, we should also consider not just how technology can act as evidence of public activity, but how it has *shaped* public activity. For instance, members of the public have actively embraced fitness trackers for personal information, sharing online and even for receiving discounts on life and health insurance (Tedesco et al. 2017). The growth of self-tracking using digital technologies has a number of significant implications for individual and collective health, and more broadly for the divide between public and private, as private information is made public, and private companies may benefit from the public's embrace of such technologies (Lupton 2016).

The global nature of such developments also has an impact on the ways in which publics are made and remade. The internet has broken down some geographic barriers while inadvertently strengthening others. For instance, vaccine hesitancy among certain 'real world' middle-class social groups has been supplemented and strengthened by anti-vaccine evidence found online and deriving from sources from around the world. Thus, pockets of unvaccinated populations have emerged in some American middle-class neighbourhoods, making cities much more vulnerable to infectious disease outbreaks than they would be if the non-vaccinated were spread more geographically evenly throughout the region (Smith et al. 2004). At the same time, public health authorities and charities have also been able to use the internet to break down taboos or find traditionally evasive publics to make interventions. For example, recent campaigns to encourage young men to seek help for depression and suicidal thoughts have relied upon the internet both for targeted advertising and as a form of confidential consultation (Campaign Against Living Miserably, n.d.; Sueki and Ito 2015). In some ways these technologies are not entirely novel—confidential telephone lines for mental health, vulnerable gay people, children, and so on, have been widespread since the 1980s (Crane and Colpus 2016)—but they have taken new forms as technology has become more mobile and more accessible in the twenty-first century.

4 Conclusion

The development of new technologies and the spaces they create for new publics is just one of the ways in which the boundaries between public and private were redrawn since 1948.

Although there was never a fixed line between 'public' and 'private' within public health, the increased emphasis on the public consequences of private behaviours blurred the boundary still further. When combined with developments outside of the public/private dichotomy that nonetheless had an impact on collective health and public health policy and practice, it is tempting to reject these distinctions as no longer of value in attempting to understand public health. Yet, public and private remain useful concepts to think with, as they draw attention to the different interest groups operating within public health and the different political strategies at work.

Archival Material

Access provided by National Survey of Health and Development, Royal College of Obstetricians and Gynaecologists and the Population Investigation Committee, 'Maternity Survey' (1946).

Parliamentary Archives HC/CP/5079, GI Grant, letter to A Milner-Barry, n.d. (probably February 1976).

Parliamentary Archives HC/CP/5059, National Dairy Council (1976) "The controversy regarding the relationship between fats and heart disease".

Parliamentary Archives HC/CP/5046, WM Dixon, letter to A Milner-Barry, 2 January 1976.

Private Collection, M Marmot to AM Semmence, 7 August 1980.

Secretary of State for Health Keith Joseph in House of Commons Debates, 19 June 1973, vol. 858, col. 380.

The National Archives, MH 154/579, Department of Health and Social Security: Proposed Survey of the number and needs of chronic sick and handicapped people. Draft paper from the Ministry of Social Security, February 1968.

Bibliography

Abbate, Janet. 2017. 'What and Where Is the Internet? (Re)Defining Internet Histories.' *Internet Histories* 1 (1–2): 8–14.

Acheson, Donald. 1998. *Independent Inquiry into Inequalities in Health*. London: The Stationary Office.

Anionwu, Elizabeth. 1988. 'Health Education and Community Development for Sickle Cell Disorders in Brent.' Institute of Education, University of London.

Anionwu, Elizabeth, and Karl Atkin. 2001. *The Politics of Sickle Cell and Thalassaemia*. Buckinghman and Phildelphia: Open University Press.

Anon, Robert. 1974. 'Can I Avoid a Heart Attack?' *The Lancet* 303 (7858): 607.

Armstrong, David. 1993. 'Public Health Spaces and the Fabrication of Identity.' *Sociology* 27 (3): 393–410.

———. 2009. 'Origins of the Problem of Health-Related Behaviours A Genealogical Study.' *Social Studies of Science* 39 (6): 909–26.

Aronowitz, Robert. 2011. 'The Framingham Heart Study and the Emergence of the Risk Factor Approach to Coronary Heart Disease, 1947–1970.' *Revue d'Histoire Des Sciences* 64 (2): 263–95.

Ashton, John, and Howard Seymour. 1988. *The New Public Health: The Liverpool Experience*. Milton Keynes: Open University Press.

Ayo, Nike. 2012. 'Understanding Health Promotion in a Neoliberal Climate and the Making of Health Conscious Citizens.' *Critical Public Health* 22 (1): 99–105.

Baggott, Rob. 2005. 'A Funny Thing Happened on the Way to the Forum? Reforming Patient and Public Involvement in the NHS in England.' *Public Administration* 83 (3): 533–51.

Baggott, Rob, and Kathryn L. Jones. 2011. 'Prevention Better Than Cure? Health Consumer and Patients' Organisations and Public Health.' *Social Science & Medicine* 73 (4): 530–34.

Baggott, Rob, Judith Allsop, and Kathryn Jones. 2005. *Speaking for Patients and Carers: Health Consumer Groups and the Policy Process.* Basingstoke: Palgrave Macmillan.

Baxter, Holly. 2013. 'Is the Internet Making You (Think You're) Ill? You're a Cyberchondriac.' *The Guardian*, 9 October 2013. https://www.theguardian.com/commentisfree/2013/oct/09/cyberchondriac-internet-ill-self-diagnose-symptoms.

Berlivet, Luc. 2005. 'Uneasy Prevention: The Problematic Modernisation of Health Education in France After 1975.' In *Medicine, the Market and the Mass Media*, edited by Virginia Berridge and Kelly Loughlin, 95–122. Abingdon: Routledge.

Berridge, Virginia. 2002. 'The Black Report and The Health Divide.' *Contemporary British History* 16 (3): 131–72.

———. 2007. *Marketing Health: Smoking and the Discourse of Public Health in Britain, 1945–2000.* Oxford: Oxford University Press.

Berridge, Virginia, and Kelly Loughlin. 2005. 'Smoking and the New Health Education in Britain 1950s–1970s.' *American Journal of Public Health* 95 (6): 956–64.

Berridge, Virginia, and Martin Gorsky. 2012. 'Introduction: Environment, Health and History.' In *Environment, Health and History*, 1–22. Basingstoke: Palgrave Macmillan.

Berridge, Virginia, and Suzanne Taylor (eds.). 2005. *The Big Smoke: Fifty Years After the 1952 London Smog.* London: Centre for History in Public Health.

Blane, David. 1985. 'An Assessment of the Black Report's Explanations of Health Inequalities.' *Sociology of Health & Illness* 7 (3): 423–45.

Blaxter, Mildred. 1983. 'Health Services as a Defence Against the Consequences of Poverty in Industrialised Societies.' *Social Science & Medicine* 17 (16): 1139–48.

Blaxter, Mildred, and E. Paterson. 1982. *Mothers and Daughters: A Three-Generational Study of Health Attitudes and Behaviour.* London: Heinemann Educational Books.

Bowcott, O. 2010. 'Cameron Is Trying to Set Out a Clear Ideological Path on the NHS'.' *The Guardian*, 5 January 2010. https://www.theguardian.com/society/joepublic/2010/jan/05/conservative-nhs-draft-manifesto.

Campaign Against Living Miserably. n.d. 'Campaign Against Living Miserably.' Accessed 6 July 2018. https://www.thecalmzone.net/.

Central Health Services Council, and Scottish Health Services Council. 1964. *Health Education.* London: HMSO.

Centre for Longditudinal Studies. n.d. 'Centre for Longitudinal Studies/Nat Cen, "Millennium Cohort Study: First Survey", (2003).' Accessed 25 July 2018a. http://www.cls.ioe.ac.uk/page.aspx?&sitesectionid=860&sitesectiontitle=Questionnaire.

———. n.d. 'Centre for Longitudinal Studies/National Birthday Trust Fund, "Perinatal Mortality Survey", (1958).' Accessed 25 July 2018b. http://www.cls.ioe.ac.uk/page.aspx?&sitesectionid=753&sitesectiontitle=Questionnaires.

———. n.d. 'CLS/National Birthday Trust Fund and the Royal College of Obstetricians and Gynaecologists, "British Births", (1970).' Accessed 25 July 2019. http://www.cls.ioe.ac.uk/page.aspx?&sitesectionid=813&sitesectiontitle=Questionnaire.

Charlton, B.G. 1995. 'A Critique of Geoffrey Rose's "Population Strategy" for Preventive Medicine.' *Journal of the Royal Society of Medicine* 88 (11): 607–10.

Clark, Christopher E., Ben Norris, A. Jayne Fordham, Maria R. Greenwood, Suzanne H. Richards, and John L. Campbell. 2018. 'Delivery and Impact of the NHS Health Check in the First 8 Years: A Systematic Review.' *British Journal of General Practice*, October. https://bjgp.org/content/delivery-and-impact-nhs-health-check-first-8-years-systematic-review.

Cm 289. 1988. *Public Health in England: The Report of the Committee of Inquiry Into the Future Development of the Public Health Function*. London: HMSO.

Connelly, Roxanne, and Lucinda Platt. 2014. 'Cohort Profile: UK Millennium Cohort Study (MCS).' *International Journal of Epidemiology* 43 (6): 1719–25.

Corton, Christine L. 2015. *London Fog: The Biography*. Cambridge: Harvard University Press.

Crane, Jennifer, and Eve Colpus. 2016. 'Childline at 30: Are Children Happier Than They Used to Be?' *The Independent*, 31 October 2016. https://www.independent.co.uk/life-style/health-and-families/features/childline-30-children-happier-mental-health-helpline-a7388951.html.

Crawford, R. 1980. 'Healthism and the Medicalization of Everyday Life.' *International Journal of Health Services: Planning, Administration, Evaluation* 10 (3): 365–88.

Crook, Tom. 2016. *Governing Systems: Modernity and the Making of Public Health in England, 1830–1910*. Oakland, CA: University of California Press.

Department of Health. 2002a. 'Department of Health, "MMR The Facts".' 8 September 2002. https://web.archive.org/web/20020908120649/http://www.mmrthefacts.nhs.uk/.

———. 2002b. 'Department of Health, "Measles, Mumps and Rubella Vaccine (MMR)".' 12 December 2002. http://web.archive.org/web/20021213092753/http:/www.doh.gov.uk/mmr/.

Department of Health and Social Security. 1976. *Prevention and Health: Everybody's Business. A Reassessment of Public and Personal Health*. London: HMSO.

Desrosières, Alain. 2010. *The Politics of Large Numbers: A History of Statistical Reasoning*, New ed. Translated by Camille Naish. Cambridge, MA: Harvard University Press.

Dorling, Danny, Richard Wilkinson, and Kate Pickett. 2015. *Injustice: Why Social Inequality Still Persists*, 2nd Rev. ed. Bristol: Policy Press.

Doyle, Y.G., A. Furey, and J. Flowers. 2006. 'Sick Individuals and Sick Populations: 20 Years Later.' *Journal of Epidemiology & Community Health* 60 (5): 396–98.

Egger, G., and B. Swinburn. 1997. 'An "Ecological" Approach to the Obesity Pandemic.' *BMJ: British Medical Journal* 315 (7106): 477–80.

Expenditure Committee. 1977. *First Report from the Expenditure Committee Together with the Minutes of Evidence Taken Before the Social Services and Employment Sub-Committee in Sessions 1975–76 and 1976–77 Appendices and Index. Preventive Medicine. Volume III. Minutes of Evidence 5th May–15th July 1976, Appendices and Index*. London: HMSO.

Færgeman, Ole. 2005. 'Commentary: Geoffrey Rose's Thinking About Coronary Artery Disease.' *International Journal of Epidemiology* 34 (2): 246–47.

Fee, Elizabeth, and Roy M. (Roy Malcolm) Acheson (eds.). 1991. *A History of Education in Public Health: Health That Mocks the Doctors' Rules*. Oxford and New York: Oxford University Press.

Forster, Rudolf, and Jonathan Gabe. 2008. 'Voice or Choice? Patient and Public Involvement in the National Health Service in England Under New Labour.' *International Journal of Health Services: Planning, Administration, Evaluation* 38 (2): 333–56.

Giroux, Élodie. 2013. 'The Framingham Study and the Constitution of a Restrictive Concept of Risk Factor.' *Social History of Medicine* 26 (1): 94–112.

Gorsky, Martin, and Gareth Millward. 2018. 'Resource Allocation for Equity in the British National Health Service, 1948–89: An Advocacy Coalition Analysis of the RAWP'. *Journal of Health Politics, Policy and Law* 43 (1): 69–108.

Gov.uk. n.d. 'Population Screening Programmes.' Accessed 24 July 2018. https://www.gov.uk/topic/population-screening-programmes.

Hampton, Jameel. 2016. *Disability and the Welfare State in Britain: Changes in Perception and Policy 1948–1979*. Bristol, UK: Policy Press.

Hand, Jane. 2017. 'Marketing Health Education: Advertising Margarine and Visualising Health in Britain from 1964–c.2000.' *Contemporary British History* 31 (4): 477–500.

Harris, Amelia I. 1971. *Handicapped and Impaired in Great Britain*. Her Majesty's Stationary Office.

Harvey, David. 2007. *A Brief History of Neoliberalism*. New ed. Oxford: Oxford University Press.

Hilton, Matthew, James McKay, Nicholas Crowson, and Jean-François Mouhot. 2013. *The Politics of Expertise: How NGOs Shaped Modern Britain*. Oxford: OUP Oxford.

Hofman, A., and J.P. Vandenbroucke. 1992. 'Geoffrey Rose's Big Idea.' *BMJ (Clinical Research Ed.)* 305 (December): 1519–20.

Hogg, Christine. 2009. *Citizens, Consumers and the NHS: Capturing Voices.* Basingstoke: Palgrave Macmillan.

Illsley, R. 1955. 'Social Class Selection and Class Differences in Relation to Stillbirths and Infant Deaths.' *British Medical Journal* 2 (4955): 1520–24.

Jackson, Mark. 2005. 'Cleansing the Air and Promoting Health: The Politics of Pollution in Postwar Britain.' In *Medicine, the Market and the Mass Media*, 221–43. Abingdon, Oxon and New York: Routledge.

Le Grand, Julian. 1978. 'The Distribution of Public Expenditure: The Case of Health Care.' *Economica* 45 (178): 125–42.

———. 2007. *The Other Invisible Hand: Delivering Public Services Through Choice and Competition.* Princeton, NJ: Princeton University Press.

Lowy, Ilana. 2011. *A Woman's Disease: The History of Cervical Cancer.* OUP Oxford.

Lupton, Deborah. 1995. *The Imperative of Health: Public Health and the Regulated Body.* London and Thousand Oaks: Sage.

———. 2016. *The Quantified Self*, 1st ed. Cambridge: Polity Press.

Macintyre, Sally. 2002. 'Before and After the Black Report: Four Fallacies.' *Contemporary British History* 16 (3): 198–220.

Marmot, Michael. 2010. 'Fair Society Healthy Lives (The Marmot Review).' http://www.instituteofhealthequity.org/resources-reports/fair-society-healthy-lives-the-marmot-review.

Marmot, Michael, G.D. Smith, S. Stansfeld, C. Patel, F. North, J. Head, I. White, E. Brunner, and A. Feeney. 1991. 'Health Inequalities Among British Civil Servants: The Whitehall II Study.' *Lancet (London, England)* 337 (8754): 1387–93.

Miller, Peter, and Nikolas Rose. 1990. 'Governing Economic Life.' *Economy and Society* 19 (1): 1–31.

Millward, Gareth. 2015. 'Social Security Policy and the Early Disability Movement—Expertise, Disability, and the Government, 1965–77.' *Twentieth Century British History* 26 (2): 274–97.

Mold, Alex. 2012. 'Patients' Rights and the National Health Service in Britain, 1960s–1980s.' *American Journal of Public Health* 102 (11): 2030–38.

———. 2013. 'Repositioning the Patient: Patient Organizations, Consumerism, and Autonomy in Britain During the 1960s and 1970s.' *Bulletin of the History of Medicine* 87 (2): 225–49.

———. 2015. *Making the Patient-Consumer: Patient Organisations and Health Consumerism in Britain.* Manchester: Manchester University Press.

———. 2017. '"Everybody Likes a Drink. Nobody Likes a Drunk". Alcohol, Health Education and the Public in 1970s Britain.' *Social History of Medicine* 30 (3): 612–36.

Morris, J.N. 1955. 'Uses of Epidemiology.' *British Medical Journal* 2 (4936): 395–401.
———. 1957. *Uses of Epidemiology*. Edinburgh and London: E&S Livingstone Ltd.
Muurinen, J.M., and J. Le Grand. 1985. 'The Economic Analysis of Inequalities in Health.' *Social Science and Medicine (1982)* 20 (10): 1029–35.
Oliver, Mike, and Jane Campbell. 1996. *Disability Politics: Understanding Our Past, Changing Our Future*, 1st ed. London and New York: Routledge.
Pearson, Helen. 2016. *The Life Project: The Extraordinary Story of Our Ordinary Lives*. London: Penguin Random House.
Petrovic, Marko, Richard Roberts, and Mary Ramsay. 2001. 'Second Dose of Measles, Mumps, and Rubella Vaccine: Questionnaire Survey of Health Professionals.' *BMJ: British Medical Journal* 322 (7278): 82–85.
Pickett, Kate, and Richard Wilkinson. 2010. *The Spirit Level: Why Equality Is Better for Everyone*. New ed. London: Penguin.
Pollock, Allyson M. 2005. *NHS Plc: The Privatisation of Our Health Care*. New Updated ed. London: Verso Books.
Porter, Dorothy. 1999. *Health, Civilization and the State: A History of Public Health from Ancient to Modern Times*. London: Routledge.
———. 2002. 'From Social Structure to Social Behaviour in Britain After the Second World War.' *Contemporary British History* 16 (3): 58–80.
———. 2007. 'Calculating Health and Social Change: An Essay on Jerry Morris and Late-Modernist Epidemiology.' *International Journal of Epidemiology* 36 (6): 1180–84.
Power, Chris, and Jane Elliott. 2006. 'Cohort Profile: 1958 British Birth Cohort (National Child Development Study).' *International Journal of Epidemiology* 35 (1): 34–41.
Prashar, Usha, and Elizabeth Anionwu. 1985. *Sickle Cell Anaemia: Who Cares? A Survey of Screening and Counselling Facilities in England*. London: Runnymede Trust.
Rodgers, search. 2012. *Age of Fracture*. Cambridge, MA: Harvard University Press.
Rose, Geoffrey. 1985. 'Sick Individuals and Sick Populations.' *International Journal of Epidemiology* 14 (1): 32–38.
———. 1992. *The Strategy of Preventive Medicine*. Oxford: Oxford University Press.
Rothstein, William G. 2003. *Public Health and the Risk Factor: A History of an Uneven Medical Revolution*. Rochester, NY: University of Rochester Press.
Salter, Brian. 2003. 'Patients and Doctors: Reformulating the UK Health Policy Community?' *Social Science & Medicine* 57 (5): 927–36.
Scott-Samuel, Alex. 1986. 'Social Inequalities in Health: Back on the Agenda.' *The Lancet* 327 (8489): 1084–85.
Selway, J. 1998. 'MMR Vaccination and Autism 1998.' *British Medical Journal* 316 (7147): 1824.

Smith, Philip J., Susan Y. Chu, and Lawrence E. Barker. 2004. 'Children Who Have Received No Vaccines: Who Are They and Where Do They Live?' *Pediatrics* 114 (1): 187–95.

Speers, Tammy, and Justin Lewis. 2004. 'Journalists and Jabs: Media Coverage of the MMR Vaccine.' *Communication & Medicine* 1 (2): 171–81.

Stern, Jon. 1983. 'Social Mobility and the Interpretation of Social Class Mortality Differentials.' *Journal of Social Policy* 12 (1): 27–49.

Stiglitz, Joseph. 2013. *The Price of Inequality*. London: Penguin.

Stott, Mary. 1989. *Forgetting's No Excuse*. New ed. London: Virago Press Ltd.

Sueki, Hajime, and Jiro Ito. 2015. 'Suicide Prevention Through Online Gate-keeping Using Search Advertising Techniques: A Feasibility Study.' *Crisis* 36 (4): 267–73.

Szreter, Simon. 2002. 'Rethinking McKeown: The Relationship Between Public Health and Social Change.' *American Journal of Public Health* 92 (5): 722–25.

Tedesco, Salvatore, John Barton, and Brendan O'Flynn. 2017. 'A Review of Activity Trackers for Senior Citizens: Research Perspectives, Commercial Landscape and the Role of the Insurance Industry.' *Sensors (Basel, Switzerland)* 17 (6): 1277.

Thorsheim, Peter. 2009. *Inventing Pollution: Coal, Smoke, and Culture in Britain since 1800*, 1st ed. Ohio University Press.

Timmermann, Carsten. 2012. 'Appropriating Risk Factors: The Reception of an American Approach to Chronic Disease in the Two German States, c. 1950–1990.' *Social History of Medicine* 25 (1): 157–74.

Townsend, Peter, Peter Davidson, and Margaret Whitehead. 1982. *Inequalities in Health: The Black Report and The Health Divide*. London: Penguin.

Turner, Fred. 2017. 'Can We Write a Cultural History of the Internet? If So, How?' *Internet Histories* 1 (1–2): 39–46.

Turner, R., and K. Ball. 1973. 'Prevention of Coronary Heart-Disease: A Counterblast to Present Inactivity.' *The Lancet* 302 (7838): 1137–40.

'UNdata | Record View | Internet Users (per 100 People)'. n.d. Accessed 22 June 2017. http://data.un.org/Data.aspx?d=WDI&f=Indicator_Code%3AIT.NET.USER.P2.

Unilever. n.d. 'Unilever Flora Pro.Activ: Test The Nation.' Accessed 25 July 2018. http://www.adeevee.com/2007/05/unilever-flora-proactiv-test-the-nation-promo/.

Vernon, James. 2017. *Modern Britain, 1750 to the Present*. Cambridge: Cambridge University Press.

Wadsworth, Michael, Diana Kuh, Marcus Richards, and Rebecca Hardy. 2006. 'Cohort Profile: The 1946 National Birth Cohort (MRC National Survey of Health and Development).' *International Journal of Epidemiology* 35 (1): 49–54.

Whitely, Paul, and Steve Winyard. 1987. *Pressure for the Poor: The Poverty Lobby and Policy Making*. London: Methuen.

Wilson, J.M.G., and G. Junger. 1968. 'Principles and Practice of Screening for Disease'. *WHO Chronicle* 22 (11): 473.

Wood, Brian. 2000. *Patient Power? The Politics of Patients' Associations in Britain and America*. Buckingham: Open University Press.

CHAPTER 6

Conclusion

Abstract In the Conclusion, we reflect on some of the important changes and continuities over time and consider the implications that these have for our understanding of the 'public' and of 'public health', now, and in the past. We do this by focusing on three areas: the place of the public in public health; the nature of public health policy and practice; and finally, the relationship between these. We locate these changes and continuities within the context of a larger debate about citizenship in post-war Britain. The multi-dimensional nature of the relationship between state and citizen within public health is just one of a number of broader implications of imagined publics and their interaction with public health.

Keywords The public · Public health · Citizenship

Since 1948, the nature of the public, public health and the relationship between these, has changed considerably. We have shown how imagined publics were brought into being by public health policymakers and practitioners, and how these publics both reflected and challenged conventional categories, identity-based or otherwise. Some of these publics, in certain circumstances, we suggested, were able to 'speak back' to public health and so alter its practice and outlook. And yet, we argue, despite all of these changes, 'publicness', as both an object and a concept, remains. What,

A. Mold et al., *Placing the Public in Public Health in Post-War Britain, 1948–2012*, Medicine and Biomedical Sciences in Modern History,
https://doi.org/10.1007/978-3-030-18685-2_6

then, has stayed the same, and what has altered? In this chapter we reflect on some of the key changes and continuities over time and consider the implications that these have for our understanding of the 'public' and of 'public health', now, and in the past. We do this by focusing on three keys areas: the place of the public in public health; the nature of public health policy and practice; and finally, the relationship between these. We locate these changes and continuities within the context of a larger debate about citizenship in post-war Britain.

1 The Place of the Public

The public had always occupied an important place within public health policy and practice but there was something different about the ways in which the public was thought of, and the actions it was required to take, in the latter part of the twentieth century. For instance, although the Victorian interest in 'habits' could be thought of as analogous with the post-war focus on 'lifestyle', there are points of departure too. From the mid-1950s onwards, individual behaviour was increasingly seen as the primary cause of disease in and of itself, not just as a way of spreading or exacerbating it. Moreover, post-war public health authorities asserted that these behaviours could be found throughout the population (albeit not evenly) and not just among the poorest. The mapping of individual disease-causing habits onto the entire population suggested a different relationship between the public and public health to what had gone before. Members of the public were expected to take on a greater role in guaranteeing their own good health and that of the collective. But, the rise of 'healthism' and the 'entrepreneurial self' can be taken too far (Crawford 1980; Miller and Rose 1990). As we demonstrate, there was still a place within public health policy and practice for thinking about and addressing external influences on health, such as social structure and the environment. Moreover, some members of the public actively rejected calls to self-manage their health.

Indeed, one consequence of a greater interest in the behaviour of the public was to bring the agency of publics into sharper focus. In the past, certain publics had agency, such as anti-vaccination groups or aggrieved rate-payers during the late nineteenth century. What was different about the agency of the public in the post-war period was the ways in which this became both an object of analysis and a tool with which to improve the public's health. Efforts to engage the public in the improvement of their own health and that of others became more important both as a way of preventing ill-health, but also as a means to cement the bond between state and citizen. At the same time, the agency of the public was not a homogenous entity. Although a greater range of publics were ascribed agency than in the past, the nature of this agency, and its interaction with questions of identity, was uneven. As we demonstrated, certain publics, such as white, middle-class men, appeared to have had more capacity to 'speak back' to public health than other, more marginalised publics, but that did not mean resistance was confined only to the most privileged groups within society. The key change, then, was not just the enhanced interest in the public and its conduct, but also the space or spaces this opened up for a variety of publics to create their own meanings and actions.

2 The Nature of Public Health

In many ways, thinking about the place of the public within public health was not a new concern for policymakers and practitioners. A long-running tension for public health authorities was how to balance the needs of the individual with those of the collective. Whether it concerned restricting personal liberty (vaccination, compulsory treatment), limiting trade (quarantine and *cordon sanitaire*) or appealing to individuals and groups to take action (health education), those working to improve the public's health were well accustomed to making trade-offs between the micro and the macro. Public health policy and practice required thinking at different levels, of the individual and the collective. One area where such multiple formulations played out was in the discourse around risk. This was not a new concept, but it did come to acquire greater significance in the thinking and practice of post-war public health than it had done previously. Risk discourse was manifested in two principle dimensions: in relation to the population, and in relation to the individual. Post-war epidemiology became increasingly concerned with the calculation and assessment of the risk of developing certain diseases among population groups. Technological changes also meant that risk calculations were increasingly sophisticated, according them greater scientific credibility. However, when this was translated into public health policy and practice, campaigns often tended to focus on the individual, and his or her risk of developing a particular condition, rather than on the whole population. This could be thought of as mirroring individualist ways of thinking about citizens and publics, but population level approaches to risk did not disappear entirely. For instance, a population level view of alcohol consumption suggested that levels of harm connected to alcohol were related to the amount of alcohol consumed within a population. In order to reduce harm, all drinkers, and not only those at significant risk of ill-health, should be encouraged to drink less (Bruun 1975). Risk, then, was of individual and collective importance, and central to many elements of post-war public health and its view of the public.

Post-war public health's focus on risk can be seen as a reflection of both the changing nature of the challenges it faced, and a shift in the outlook of those involved in public health policy and practice. The impact that these changes had on the public health 'system' are hard to disentangle from other developments. As Tom Crook points out, public health 'systems' were complex and dynamic in the early part of the twentieth century, but there is a good case to be made that these became even more complex and dynamic as the century progressed. The widening of public health authorities' gaze to include more of the everyday lives of ordinary people meant that an even broader range of behaviours, settings and activities could be considered within the compass of 'public health'. At the same time, as the state was 'rolled back' from many areas of health and welfare provision, the variety of actors involved in ensuring good public health increased. 'Who' public health authorities were became harder to discern as 'what' public health consisted of broadened.

3 The Relationship Between the Public and Public Health

The relationship between the public and public health did not play out in isolation from other developments. Indeed, this can be seen as an exemplar of the fluctuating interaction between the state and citizen. The precise kinds of citizenship operating within post-war public health can be broken into three categories: hygienic, social and consumer. Hygienic citizenship was about modernity, order and standards of behaviour, especially, but not only, related to cleanliness. It was a concept identified by historians interested in public health during the late nineteenth and early twentieth century particularly in the colonial context (Anderson 2006; Bashford 2003). But hygienic citizenship was applied at home too, in both the inter- and post-war periods (Welshman 1997; Bivins 2015). This can be seen, for instance, in the continued interest by Medical Officers of Health in food hygiene and domestic cleanliness throughout the 1950s and into the 1960s (Mold 2018). Personal hygiene was also a key element of health education efforts that aimed to promote morality and good citizenship in the immediate post-war decades. Hygienic citizenship was, to some extent, a hangover from the pre-bacteriological revolution era, when cleanliness was required in order to prevent the spread of disease. However, the emphasis on health as both a personal responsibility and collective duty can be found in other, later, formulations of public health citizenship too.

The balance between individual rights and collective responsibilities was central to notions of social citizenship. According to the key authority on social citizenship, T. H. Marshall, social rights permitted the citizen access to a minimum supply of essential social goods and services (such as medical attention, shelter and education), to be provided by the state (Marshall 1992). The NHS, and the other achievements of the 'classic' era of the British welfare state (from 1945 to 1975), appeared to offer a kind of social citizenship based on collective rights. Social citizenship was rooted in pre and immediate post-war ideas of social medicine. Dorothy Porter suggests that social medicine was the means through which health could be included in Marshall's social rights on which citizenship in the 1950s would be based. But, she argues, such ideals were rapidly undermined. From the mid-1950s onwards, social medicine became less concerned with the impact of social structure on health, and more concerned with individual behaviour (Porter 2002). Yet, as we pointed to throughout this book, ideas about collective and individual rights and responsibilities did not go away within public health policy and practice, nor did they disappear within public understandings of health.

Nonetheless, by the late 1970s, social citizenship as an organising concept appeared to be being eroded by consumer citizenship. Consumerism as applied to health was about a set of ideas and policies orientated around autonomy, representation, complaint, rights, information and choice (Mold 2015). Of all of these, it is choice that is most often associated with consumerism, and the value that seems to have frequently trumped all the others. Choice did feature in public health policy and practice, particularly in health education campaigns that emphasised the need to make 'healthy choices' (Hand 2017). Yet, this progressive narrative, of one form of citizenship replacing another, can be upset. Elements of hygienic citizenship persisted, and indeed were reborn in the wake of the HIV/AIDS epidemic (Armstrong 1993). Social citizenship continues to underpin many collective efforts to ensure good health. Consumer citizenship was not entirely unique to this period, and, we argue, nor did it totally crowd out other forms of citizenship. Just as there are many publics, so too there are many different ways of thinking about individuals and their relationship to and with the state (Grant 2016).

One example of the overlapping of various forms of citizenship can be seen in the public health survey. In the immediate post-war period, public health surveyors relied on individuals' sense of public duty to garner enough respondents. This notion of duty was based on the post-war social contract, which emphasised responsibilities as well as rights. The right to access to public services, like education and healthcare, was balanced with responsibilities such as using these in a rational manner. Many would argue that this form of social citizenship held until the 1970s, when the welfare state, and the values which underpinned it, came under attack. The emergence of more individuated approaches to public services (whether these be termed 'neoliberal', 'consumerist' or 'entrepreneurial') led to a shift in the types of surveys being conducted and the actions of the surveyed population. Public opinion, for instance, came to matter more, as an object to be surveyed and as something to be taken into account when designing public health policies. However, that did not mean that 'publicness' disappeared. Surveyors still found willing subjects, and collective responsibility had not been eclipsed entirely by individual choice.

The multi-dimensional nature of the relationship between state and citizen within public health is just one of a number of broader implications of imagined publics and their interaction with public health. For historians and social scientists, we suggest that our analysis highlights the dynamic processes that go in to making up people and practices, and that these are not unidirectional. Similarly, for public health practitioners today, it is important to recognise that there has long been and continues to be a multiplicity of publics, and these should be allowed to speak, even if what they are saying is sometimes hard to hear.

Bibliography

Anderson, Warwick. 2006. *Colonial Pathologies: American Tropical Medicine, Race, and Hygiene in the Philippines.* London and Durham: Duke University Press.

Armstrong, David. 1993. Public Health Spaces and the Fabrication of Identity. *Sociology* 27 (3): 393–410.

Bashford, A. 2003. *Imperial Hygiene: A Critical History of Colonialism, Nationalism and Public Health.* 2004 ed. Houndmills, Basingstoke and New York: Palgrave Macmillan.

Bivins, Roberta E. 2015. *Contagious Communities: Medicine, Migration, and the NHS in Post-war Britain.* Oxford: Oxford University Press.

Bruun, Kettil. 1975. *Alcohol Control Policies in Public Health Perspective.* The Finnish Foundation for Alcohol Studies. New Brunswick, NJ: Distributors, Rutgers University Center of Alcohol Studies.

Crawford, R. 1980. 'Healthism and the Medicalization of Everyday Life.' *International Journal of Health Services: Planning, Administration, Evaluation* 10 (3): 365–88.

Grant, Matthew. 2016. Historicizing Citizenship in Post-war Britain. *The Historical Journal* 59 (4): 1187–1206.

Hand, Jane. 2017. Marketing Health Education: Advertising Margarine and Visualising Health in Britain from 1964–c.2000. *Contemporary British History* 31 (4): 477–500.

Marshall, T.H. 1992. 'Citizenship and Social Class.' In *Citizenship and Social Class.* London: Pluto Press.

Miller, Peter, and Nikolas Rose. 1990. Governing Economic Life. *Economy and Society* 19 (1): 1–31.

Mold, Alex. 2015. *Making the Patient-Consumer: Patient Organisations and Health Consumerism in Britain.* Manchester: Manchester University Press.

———. 2018. 'Exhibiting Good Health: Public Health Exhibitions in London, 1948–71.' *Medical History* 62 (1): 1–26.

Porter, Dorothy. 2002. From Social Structure to Social Behaviour in Britain After the Second World War. *Contemporary British History* 16 (3): 58–80.

Welshman, John. 1997. "Bringing Beauty and Brightness to the Back Streets": Health Education and Public Health in England and Wales, 1890–1940. *Health Education Journal* 56 (2): 199–209.

Index

A. Mold et al., *Placing the Public in Public Health in Post-War Britain 1948-2012*, Medicine and Biomedical Sciences in Modern History,
https://doi.org/10.1007/978-3-030-18685-2

www.ingramcontent.com/pod-product-compliance
Lightning Source LLC
LaVergne TN
LVHW082237200926
848484LV00008B/2366
9781013276453